T0073458

ACUPUNCTURE
Theories and Evidence

ACUPUNCTURE

Theories and Evidence

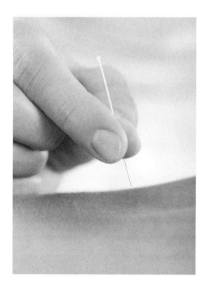

Editor

HONG Hai

Nanyang Technological University, Singapore

World Scientific

NEW JERSEY · LONDON · SINGAPORE · BEIJING · SHANGHAI · HONG KONG · TAIPEI · CHENNAI

Published by

World Scientific Publishing Co. Pte. Ltd.

5 Toh Tuck Link, Singapore 596224

USA office: 27 Warren Street, Suite 401-402, Hackensack, NJ 07601

UK office: 57 Shelton Street, Covent Garden, London WC2H 9HE

Library of Congress Cataloging-in-Publication Data
Acupuncture : theories and evidence / edited by Hong Hai.
    p. ; cm.
    Includes bibliographical references and index.
    ISBN 978-9814452014 (hardcover : alk. paper)
    I. Hong, Hai, 1943–
    [DNLM: 1. Acupuncture. WB 369]
    615.8'92--dc23
                        2012046516

British Library Cataloguing-in-Publication Data
A catalogue record for this book is available from the British Library.

Typeset by Stallion Press
Email: enquiries@stallionpress.com

Printed in Singapore by B & Jo Enterprise Pte Ltd

CONTENTS

PRINCIPAL CONTRIBUTORS*

Bian Zhaoxiang
Director, Clinical Division and Associate Dean, School of Chinese Medicine, Hong Kong Baptist University (BA Nanjing University of TCM, Master of Medicine, Beijing University of Chinese Medicine, PhD Guangzhou University of TCM)

Professor Bian previously served as a lecturer and Associate Professor at Guangzhou University of Traditional Chinese Medicine. He was awarded the National Science and Technology Award (2nd Class) in 2001, and the President award of Hong Kong Baptist University in 2005. He is an honorary Professor of Tianjin University of Traditional Chinese Medicine and Chinese Academy of Chinese Medical Sciences. His research focuses on the basic mechanism of visceral pain and gastrointestinal motility disorder; pharmacological effects of Chinese medicine formulas on chronic diseases, clinical trial design for Chinese medicines, and drug development for gastrointestinal disorders.

Stephen Birch
Associate Professor at the University College of Health Science — Campus Kristiania, Department of Acupuncture, Oslo (PhD in acupuncture research)

*Only the principal authors who delivered the papers at the symposium have been listed here. Chinese names listed here follow the traditional convention of placing the family name first.

Professor Stephen Birch has been practicing acupuncture since 1982 and specializes in Japanese acupuncture. He is also the senior instructor in Europe for Manaka's system 'yin-yang channel balancing therapy' and co-author of Manaka's book 'Chasing the Dragon's Tail'. He has authored six other books and many papers on acupuncture. He is the founding president of the Stichting Foundation for the Study of Traditional East Asian Medicine and founding past president of the Society for Acupuncture Research (SAR).

Edzard Ernst

Emeritus Professor, University of Exeter; Professor in Physical Medicine and Rehabilitation (PMR) at Hannover Medical School (Germany) and Head of the PMR Department at the University of Vienna (Austria)

Professor Ernst qualified as a physician in Germany where he also completed his MD and PhD theses. He arrived at the University of Exeter in 1993 to establish the first Chair in Complementary Medicine. He is founder/Editor-in-Chief of the medical journals *FACT* (Focus on Alternative and Complementary Therapies) and *Perfusion*. His has been awarded with 14 scientific prizes/awards. He served on the Medicines Commission of the British 'Medicines and Healthcare Products Regulatory Agency' (1994–2005) and on the 'Scientific Committee on Herbal Medicinal Products' of the Irish Medicines Board. In 1999 he took British nationality. He has published more than 1000 papers in the peer-reviewed literature. Blogs: BMJ, Pulse, Guardian.

Dylan Evans

Psychology Department, American University of Beirut (PhD in Philosophy, London School of Economics)

Dr Evans is the founder of Projection Point, the global leader in risk intelligence solutions. He is the author of several popular books, including *Placebo: Mind over matter in Modern Medicine, Risk Intelligence: How to Live with Uncertainty,* and *Emotion: The Science of Sentiment.* He has held academic appointments at King's College London, the University of Bath, and the American University of Beirut. He is a Distinguished Supporter of the British Humanist Association.

Hong Hai

Senior Fellow, Institute of Advanced Studies and Adjunct Professor, Nanyang Technological University (MPhil Cambridge in Philosophy of Science, MD Beijing University of Chinese Medicine)

Professor Hong Hai is a Singapore-licensed TCM physician. He previously served on the TCM Practitioners Board and was Chairman of the board's Academic Committee. Educated originally in engineering, he subsequently completed graduate studies in economics, Chinese medicine, and the philosophy of science. He has published in various Chinese medical journals and recently co-authored the book *Cancer Management with Chinese Medicine*. He practises part-time at the Public Free Clinic and the Renhai Clinic (*www.renhaitang.com.sg*). His primary research interest is in the theory of Chinese medicine from the perspective of Western philosophy of science. He serves on the editorial board of the *American Journal of Chinese Medicine.*

Hsieh Ching-Liang

Professor and Director, Graduate Institute of Integrated Medicine, China Medical University, and Director, Center for Clinical Trials in Chinese Medicine, China Medical University Hospital, Taichung, Taiwan. (PhD in Medical Science, Kyushu University, Japan, PhD in Acupuncture and Moxibustion Massage, Guangzhou Chinese Medicine University)

Professor Hsieh is a director of the International Society of Oriental Medicine and serves on the editorial board of *Evidence-Based Complementary and Alternative Medicine* and *ISRN Pain*. He holds practising licenses in both Western and Chinese medicine. He has published over one hundred papers on topics ranging from basic physiology and clinical research in acupuncture to the effect of TCM on stroke and epilepsy. He was formerly director, School of Chinese Medicine, Graduate China Medical University and Professor, Chang Gung University.

Lao Lixing

Professor of Family Medicine and the Director of Traditional Chinese Medicine Research Program, Centre for Integrative Medicine, University of Maryland (BMed Shanghai University of TCM, PhD in Physiology, University of Maryland)

A licensed acupuncturist, Prof Lao has practiced acupuncture and Chinese herbal medicine for 30 years and previously served as a board member of the Maryland State Board of Acupuncture. He is principal investigator and co-investigator of a number of clinical trials and pre-clinical studies in acupuncture and Chinese herbal medicine funded by the National Institutes of Health and US Department of Defence. He is particularly interested in conducting translational research that bridges basic science, clinical trials, and "real world" acupuncture clinical practice. He has published over 130 peer-reviewed scientific papers and over 40 non-peer reviewed invited papers and book chapters. Professor Lao was a board member of the *Society for Acupuncture Research (SAR)* and has served as a co-president of the *SAR*. He is an associate editor in the *Journal of Alternative and Complementary Medicine,* the *Journal of Chinese Medicine.*

Lee Tat Leang

Professor and senior consultant, Department of Anaesthesia, National University Health System, Singapore; clinical director of acupuncture service at the National University Hospital (MBBS, Master of Medicine (Anaesthesia) National University of Singapore, Fellow of the Australian and New Zealand College of Anaesthetists, Certificate in acupuncture and moxibustion, Chinese Academy of TCM)

Professor Lee has serrved on the Chinese Proprietary Medicine Advisory Committee (Chairman), Medicinal Advisory Committee, Specialist Accreditation Board, TCM Practitioners Board, and the Scientific Review Committee on Claims of Complementary and Alternative Medicine. He is a past president of the Singapore Society of Anaesthesiologists and has been a member of the editorial boards of *Anesthesia and Analgesia, Pain Practice, Acta Anaesthesiologica Taiwanica, Journal of Acupuncture and Tuina Science,* and *Evidence-Based Complementary and Alternative Medicine.* In 2011, he was awarded the long service medal in recognition of his contribution to the National University of Singapore and the National Outstanding Clinician Mentor Award by the Ministry of Health.

Leung Ping Chung

Professor of Orthopaedics & Traumatology, Faculty of Medicine; Director of Centre for Clinical Trials on Chinese Medicine; Chairman, Management Committee, Institute of Chinese Medicine, The Chinese University of Hong Kong (OBE, JP, Hon DSSc, DSC, MBBS, MS, FRACS, FRCS(Edin), FHKCOS, FHKAM(Orth))

Prof Leung's research areas include orthopaedics, osteoporosis, microsurgery health, and TCM. He is the author of over 600 scientific manuscripts in journals and 27 books. Publications in Chinese medicine include: *A Comprehensive Guide to Chinese Medicine* and "Treatment of Low Back Pain with Acupuncture". As Chairman of the Management Committee of the Institute of Chinese Medicine in Hong Kong, Prof Leung has contributed to modernizing Traditional Chinese Medicine. Currently, there are more than 30 clinical trials research projects underway at the Institute of Chinese Medicine. Notable international collaborations include NIH grants with Harvard University the Memorial Sloan Kettering Cancer Centre, and CNRS of France.

Thomas Lundeberg

Senior consultant in Rehabilitation Medicine University, Stockholm at Danderyds Hospital and Karolinska Hospital Huddinge (MD Karolinska Institutet, PhD in Physiology Institute of Neurobiology)

Professor Lundeberg started teaching in Karolinska Institutet before becoming Professor in Pain and Sensory Physiology. Thereafter he started to work at Karolinska Hospital as a senior consultant in Physical Medicine and Rehabilitation. He is the editor-in-chief of ARTE. He was previously Head, Section of Integrative Sensory Physiology and Chief of Medical Services, Section of Alternative Medicine, at the Karolinska Institute. He is the author of over 300 papers in scientific peer reviewed journals including and has supervised more than 10 doctoral dissertations at the Karolinska Institute. His extensive research collaborations include projects in with Australia, the Czech Republic, Great Britain, Italy and Japan.

Konstantina Theodoratou

President of the Scientific Association of Medical Acupuncture, Greece (M.D., MSc, Med. Psyc. National University of Athens, Master in Acupuncture, Guangzhou University of Chinese Medicine)

Dr Konstantina Theodoratou undertook her medical studies in Athens, Beijing and Tianjin and went on to further her studies in Guangzhou University of Chinese Medicine. She has been practising acupuncture since 1996 and has taught at various programs such as Scientific Association of Medical Acupuncture in Greece, Research Institute of Acupuncture in North Greece and Hellenic Veterinary Medical Society. She is currently working on research in medical acupuncture at the Guangzhou University of Chinese Medicine.

Zhang Zhang-Jin

Associate Professor and Assistant Director (Clinical Affairs), School of Chinese Medicine, University of Hong Kong. (BMed Shanghai University of TCM, PhD in neuroscience Jiaotong University College of Medicine).

Professor Zhang was Vice-chairman of Department of Human Anatomy in Xi'an Jiaotong University College of Medicine before moving in 1996 to the USA to research in psychopharmacology and neuropsychiatry at Vanderbilt University and the Uniformed Services University of the Health Sciences, returning to Hong Kong in 2006. His long-term research interest is to develop novel therapeutic agents and alternative treatment strategies particularly using Chinese medicine and acupuncture for major neuropsychiatric disorders. He has authored and co-authored over 60 peer-reviewed papers and 5 book chapters. He obtained certificates as an Acupuncturist and Herbalist from National Certification Commission for Certificate for Acupuncture and Oriental Medicine of USA in 1998 and currently has an active clinical practice in Hong Kong, focusing on major neuropsychiatric disorders.

FOREWORD

Acupuncture is widely practised in clinics and hospitals throughout the developed world. But is it based on science, and is there clear evidence that it works?

These burning questions were vigorously debated at the International Symposium on Theory and Evidence in Acupuncture held from August 21–22, 2012 at Nanyang Technological University, Singapore. This volume contains 12 scientific papers by some of the world's leading researchers in acupuncture. The authors represented such internationally diverse institutions with research interests in Chinese medicine as China Medical University (Taiwan), Exeter University (UK), Hong Kong University, Karolinska Institute (Sweden), National University of Singapore and University of Maryland. They offer contrasting biomedical explanations for its action and critically examine clinical evidence for its alleged efficacy as a medical intervention for the treatment of pain and a variety of other common ailments.

Discussion sessions among panel speakers with active audience participation were engaging and thought-provoking even if no firm final conclusions were reached. These papers will undoubtedly stimulate more in-depth research into the science of acupuncture and how it can play a role in modern healthcare.

The symposium attracted a wide audience, including medical doctors, Chinese medical practitioners and academic researchers. On behalf of the Institute of Advanced Studies, I wish to thank the many individuals who contributed to it. These include Dr Amy Khor, Minister of State for Health and Manpower who graced the opening ceremony, Professors Ng Han

Seong and Hong Hai who chaired the discussion sessions, the symposium organizing committee chaired by Professors Hew Choy Sin and Kwek Leong Chuan with advisors Professors Hong Hai and Leung Ping-Chung, and the staff of IAS who worked tirelessly to make the symposium a success.

Professor Phua Kok Khoo
Director
The Institute of Advanced Studies
Nanyang Technological University
Singapore

INTRODUCTION

Hong Hai

Senior Fellow, Institute of Advanced Studies and
Adjunct Professor, Nanyang Technological University, Singapore

Kipling's lament, "Oh, East is East and West is West, and never the twain shall meet", has been superseded by acupuncture.

Ever since President Nixon's historic visit to China in 1972, when American scientists in Beijing watched with wonder acupuncture in action, and the publication of *Celestial Lancets* in 1980 by Lu Gwei-Djen and Joseph Needham at Cambridge, there has been an impressive proliferation of this ancient Eastern medical practice in the Western world. Acupuncture is now widely practised in developed Western countries. Most states in the US have licensing boards for acupuncturists and allow medical insurance claims for acupuncture and related interventions.

There has also been an explosion of research in acupuncture. But after over forty years of research and debate, the jury is still out over the question: "How does it work, and does it really work?" These direct and basic questions do not have simple answers, as the 12 scientific papers in this volume presented recently at an international symposium in Singapore amply demonstrate. The intellectual gap in the debate is not between East and West. Acupuncture is used throughout most of the developed Western world for the treatment of pain as well as a variety of ailments ranging from indigestion to impotence. But neither the mechanism of its action nor its efficacy as a medical intervention has been conclusively demonstrated by scientific studies. Explanations for the mechanism of its action depends on which acupuncture is done, whether it is the traditional Chinese method based on meridian system, or various others, including Japanese and Western methods. On clinical trials, few doubt that as an intervention it has therapeutic effects comparable to or exceeding those of standard care. The scientific question concerns how it achieves this therapeutic effect. While there is growing consensus that the placebo effect looms large in most acupuncture interventions, there remains a great divergence of opinion over whether it is the main effect, or even the *only* significant effect.

MECHANISMS

Lundeberg's paper "Mechanisms of acupuncture in pain" explains that needle stimulation represents the artificial activation of systems obtained by natural biological effects. Sensory stimulation triggers fundamental physiological changes by exciting receptors and or nerve fibers in the stimulated tissue similar to those physiologically activated by strong muscle contractions. The effects on certain organ functions are also similar to those obtained by protracted exercise. On the other hand light superficial needling, as often used during 'sham' acupuncture, excites cutaneous touch receptors, resulting in a limbic 'touch response' with a suggested role in well-being and social bonding. Lundberg argues that the effects of acupuncture in pain cannot be explained by one mechanism, as pain itself is not a physiological entity, but a multitude of varying neuroplastic changes that are part of adaptive or maladaptive reactions.

Birch raises questions regarding traditionally-based systems of acupuncture (TBSAs): How are they different from other styles of acupuncture? What are the assumptions about the nature of things that underlie TBSAs? How is this thinking different from the assumptions about the nature of things that underlie modern scientific knowledge of the world? Birch explores these issues in relation to the notion of the 'explanatory' models underlying TBSAs and biomedical knowledge of the body and examines the impact of these differences on how we develop testable 'explanatory models' of TBSAs.

In acupuncture we find three kinds of 'explanatory' models, the first a mechanistic one, the second based on known physiology and the third derived from traditional qi-based descriptions of the body. The first arises out of research on a particular clinical outcome. For example if acupuncture is said to reduce pain, what mechanisms must or could be involved for the therapy to be able to reduce the pain? The second explanatory model utilises known physiological entities and their pathways of action. This kind of explanatory model proposes that acupuncture works through those entities, for example, that acupuncture points are trigger points. This kind of model is developed by replacing the original concepts of acupuncture with more plausible sounding established biomedical concepts (replacement models). The third type of explanatory model developed as acupuncture began developing in the period 150–100 BCE and is used by TBSAs. They make reference to concepts such as qi, jingmai (meridians), xue 穴 (acu-holes), needling to regulate *qi*, xu-shi (deficiency-excess), and bu-xie 补泻 (strengthen-drain).

Hong's "Ontological status of meridians" points out that the traditional Chinese medicine (TCM) explanation of acupuncture, on the other hand, draws largely on the meridian system comprising a complex network of passages that transports *qi*, blood, and *jing* throughout the body. This system is alleged to connect the vital organs among themselves and links them to all other parts of the body, allowing the body to function as an organic whole. But in the light of the modern TCM concept of the organs as a set of functions rather than somatic structures with fixed loci, the notion of meridians as physical paths leading to organs becomes suspect. Conventional meridian maps, showing the intricate paths of each meridian leading to an endpoint in a (Western anatomy) organ, would conceivably come to grief. An alternative explanation of the meridian system is that body has been observed to behave *as if* these discrete pathways exist, and organ functioning can be regulated through stimulating points on these pathways. We then treat this presumed existence as a convenient tool for locating of acupoints for needling. The philosophical issue shifts from one of ontology to that of the scientifically verifiable efficacy of treatments using these pathways as a guide for choosing the points.

Hsieh takes a more traditional Chinese view of acupuncture theory. To him, acupuncture at a certain point produces a moderating action to correct imbalances between *yin* and *yang* or between *qi* and blood. Each point has its own specific function, and the acupuncturist treats disease through a combination of needle manipulation and points. Hsieh contends that protocols and modern medical devices used to verify traditional acupuncture theory indicate that (1) acupuncture at the points of spleen and liver meridians induce a change in the mean blood flow or perfusion in the liver and spleen, implying that the meridian system does connect to both a specific internal organ and joint; (2) acupuncture at the left and right Waiguan (TE5) points induces a change in red blood velocity of nail-fold microcirculation, suggesting the ongoing interplay of circulation of qi and blood in the meridian; (3) manual acupuncture or 2 Hz electroacupuncture (EA) at both Zusanli (ST36) increases the amplitude of the P25 component of median nerve short-latency somatosensory evoked potential; it also prolongs the latency and decreases the amplitude of the sympathetic skin response suggesting that acupuncture can modulate and correct imbalances; (4) 2 Hz and 100 Hz EA at Zusanli induces a decrease in pulse rate, demonstrating the specificity of points; and (5) 2 Hz EA applied to both Zusanli and Shangjuxu (ST37) points increases the natural logarithmic high-frequency (InHF) component of heart rate viability (HRV), whereas 15 Hz EA increased InLF of HRV. These findings, overall, "provide at least partial modern scientific evidence to support the theory of traditional acupuncture".

Theodoratou approaches the problem from the viewpoint of cognitive neuroscience and acupuncture as a widely-accepted effective treatment for acute and chronic pain. During the last decades our understanding of the way the brain processes acupuncture analgesia has developed considerably with imaging technologies like fMRI and PET applied to the brains of people experiencing pain. They indicate that acupuncture controls pain by making specific brain cells more sensitive to the pain-dampening effects of opioid chemicals. Pain is a universal phenomenon with complex biochemical, neural and psychological components. The pain matrix is a multi-faceted brain network that processes painful experiences through its multiple nociceptive and anti-nociceptive pathways. The human brain has the ability not only to receive and perceive our surroundings, but also to manipulate the way in which we perceive them. Cognitive neuroscience and neuropsychology, connecting the mind and body, study the same brain activity, having to do with the transmission, interpretation and, ultimately, the very perception of pain. Cognition can alter both pain perception and acupuncture treatment effectiveness. Theodoratou reports an ongoing study into the way our mind and brain manipulate our perception of pain and control the effect of acupuncture treatment.

CLINICAL TRIALS

The more pragmatic and pressing question concerns the real clinical effects of acupuncture. Ernst laments in "Frequent weaknesses in acupuncture trials" that many RCTs have been burdened with major flaws and relatively few RCTs are low in the risk of bias and confounding factors. Some do not even have non-acupuncture controls or control for placebo effects. In his view, the influence of the therapist is an important potential confounder in acupuncture studies, and while it is clearly not easy to blind acupuncturists in clinical trials, very few investigators have even attempted to incorporate this feature in their studies. In Ernst's experience, a much deeper and more intractable problem for acupuncture research is the researcher himself. By and large, this community consists of "enthusiastic amateurs who tend to use science to prove that their prior beliefs are correct rather than to rigorously test hypotheses". When testing hypotheses, scientists conventionally conduct experiment after experiment aimed at testing whether their initial idea was wrong. If, at the end, they fail to show that the hypothesis was false, they assume that it is probably correct. Unfortunately, Ernst asserts, this process of falsification of hypotheses has not been adopted by many acupuncture researchers.

The findings of Bian *et al.* from a meta-analysis of RCTs on acupuncture did not fundamentally disagree with Ernst's dim view of the quality of such clinical trials. A search of the OVID and EMBASE database was conducted to identify the articles of RCTs with acupuncture for the low back pain. A revised CONSORT checklist and STRICTA checklist, containing 78 items with 23 items specifically for acupuncture, was applied to assess the quality of the reporting. Forty four articles on RCTs met requirements. The overall reporting quality of the RCTs of acupuncture which were assessed this way varied between 19% and 70%, with a median score of 43%. The authors also examined various designs of sham acupuncture, comprising superficial needling on acupuncture points, non-specific needling control, non-insertion simulated needling control and transcutaneous electrical nerve stimulation. Their conclusion is that the overall reporting quality of RCTs of acupuncture is low and that control design of acupuncture also needs improvement.

Lao and Zhang have a more sanguine view of acupuncture research conducted in recent years, opining that while the current research is not without its problems and difficulties, the acupuncture research community has matured and developed better research methodologies and applied new technologies, and are engaging in more creative and innovative translational research. However challenging problems remain, mainly due to the nature of acupuncture practice and the inherent differences between acupuncture and Western medicine. In clinical pharmaceutical research, the mechanism of action of a drug is often clear long before the drug reaches the clinical trial stage, and a placebo tablet lacking that mechanism can be designed and employed. Since acupuncture's mechanisms of actions are still largely unknown, it is not easy to identify a sham procedure that does not have actions similar to those of real acupuncture. Moreover, 'sham acupuncture' is poorly defined in terms of location and manipulation. Reported sham procedures include non-needle insertion, shallow insertion at non-acupuncture points, and the use of acupuncture points that are irrelevant for a given condition. Sham procedures such as needle insertion may induce non-specific physiological changes that play a more important role than a simple placebo effect. Furthermore, the existing evidence shows that the most challenging issue in acupuncture trial design is choice of an appropriate control group. Because many factors may profoundly determine therapeutic outcome, the so-called negative outcomes produced by some randomized controlled trials might actually be false negatives due to non-specific responses induced by the control.

Focusing on chronic low back pain as among the most common complaints for acupuncture intervention, Lee and Zheng compare clinical trials through tests that establish the overall *effectiveness* of the intervention against those that test its *efficacy*. The typical efficacy question would be, "How efficacious is acupuncture in the treatment of chronic low back pain as compared to sham acupuncture or no acupuncture?" (Explanatory trial on efficacy). A question on effectiveness on the other hand would be, "How effective is acupuncture in the treatment of chronic low back pain as compared to pharmacotherapy?" (Pragmatic trial on effectiveness). Effective and adequate treatment is an important issue for patients, clinicians and policy makers. In one RCT involving 230 patients reported in U K, acupuncture care was significantly more effective in reducing bodily pain than usual care at the 24-month follow-up. In addition, the acupuncture service was found to be cost-effective at 24 months. In view of the complex pathophysiology of many chronic pain conditions, the lack of a credible sham control, and a strong placebo effect associated with the use of invasive technique, Lee and Zheng consider that the differences between efficacy and effectiveness studies reflect the differences in assessing the components of acupuncture or the whole effect of acupuncture. Instead, they recommend that we should concentrate on doing more pragmatic studies focusing on the effectiveness and to include additional aspects of the traditional diagnosis on various types of chronic pain conditions. The authors also cite a study suggesting that in the current cost-conscious environment, policy makers put effectiveness above efficacy. This may represent a societal shift toward 'patient-centered health care' and away from the 'evidence-based medicine' of researchers for determining an intervention's legitimacy.

The placebo effect in acupuncture is examined by Dylan, in particular the implications of the choice of placebo for (1) proper blinding, and (2) the nature of the hypothesis being tested in any given trial. The role of placebos in clinical trials of acupuncture raises two important problems. First, the difficulty of constructing a placebo that ensures double blinding in acupuncture trials means that when such trials show acupuncture to be more effective than the placebo, the most obvious explanation is that the placebo response is activated more intensely by real acupuncture than by the sham version. The result is that acupuncture seems better than a placebo only when the condition being treated is, in fact, placebo responsive. Second, the choice of placebo will also depend on one's theory about how acupuncture is supposed to work. If this theory specifies that needles must be placed accurately at points on various meridians, then the Park Sham Device may be appropriate, but if this theory specifies that the skin must be penetrated, then this device will not be suitable. It may be that these details have not been made sufficiently explicit by the proponents of acupuncture, in which case the debate about suitable placebos for use in acupuncture trials might provide a useful opportunity for acupuncturists to develop their theories in more detail.

The last two papers in this volume deal with interesting applications of acupuncture and acupuncture-related treatments for non-pain conditions.

Leung *et al.* review literature on acupuncture treatment for withdrawal symptoms of heroin addicts which claims very positive results. A pilot study on auricular acupressure as an anti-smoking intervention and an aid with the relief of withdrawal symptoms showed that although there was a lack of statistical evidence to support the efficacy of the active treatment, both active and sham groups revealed a large reduction in the number of cigarettes consumed, confirmed by a substantial reduction of the carbon monoxide level in the breathing tests. The authors conclude that although acupressure on the external auricle is a simple maneuver, the positive results reached promising levels, taking acupoints and sham points together. The authors suggest that acupressure is a safe technique for helping smokers to quit, applicable also to pregnant and breastfeeding women for whom nicotine replacement therapy might not be as safe.

Zhang and Man report results from trials on dense cranial electroacupuncture stimulation (DCEAS), a novel stimulation mode in which electrical stimulation is delivered on dense acupoints located on the forehead mainly innervated by the trigeminal nerve. Neuroanatomical evidence suggests that, compared to the spinal-supraspinal pathways, the trigeminal sensory pathway has much intimate connections with the brainstem reticular formation, particularly the dorsal raphe nucleus (DRN) and the locus coeruleus (LC), both of which are the major resources of serotonergic (5-HT) and noradrenergic neuronal bodies respectively and play a pivotal role in the regulation of sensation, emotion, sleep, and cognition processing. This led to the hypothesis that direct stimulation on forehead acupoints in the trigeminal territory could more efficiently produce therapeutic response in neuropsychiatric disorders. Several pilot studies have shown the benefit of DCEAS and similar interventions in patients with headache, refractory obsessive-compulsive disorder (OCD), postpartum depression, and insomnia. A more recent study suggests the effectiveness of DCEAS as an additional therapy in the early-phase treatment of depression.

PART I

SCIENTIFIC EXPLANATIONS FOR ACUPUNCTURE

MECHANISMS OF ACUPUNCTURE IN PAIN: A PHYSIOLOGICAL PERSPECTIVE IN A CLINICAL CONTEXT

Thomas Lundeberg

Karolisnka Institutet, Solna, Stockholm County, Sweden

Abstract

Acupuncture is part of Traditional Chinese Medicine, a medical system with an empirical basis. A lack of scientific studies to prove the claimed effects of acupuncture has led to its rejection by many of the Western scientific community. Now that the mechanisms can be partly explained in terms of endogenous mechanisms, and the reported effects are similar or sometimes even superior to established treatments, the integration of acupuncture with conventional medicine may be possible. The effects of acupuncture are likely to devolve from physiological and/or psychological mechanisms with biological foundations, and the needle stimulation could represent the artificial activation of systems obtained by natural biological effects in functional situations. Acupuncture and some other forms of sensory stimulation trigger similar effects in man and other mammals, suggesting that they bring about fundamental physiological changes. Acupuncture stimulation, eliciting 'de qi', excites receptors and or nerve fibers in the stimulated tissue, which are also similarly physiologically activated by strong muscle contractions. The effects on certain organ functions are also similar to those obtained by protracted exercise. On the other hand light superficial needling, as often used during 'sham' acupuncture, excites cutaneous touch receptors resulting in a limbic 'touch response' with a suggested role in wellbeing and social bonding. The effects of acupuncture in pain cannot be explained by one mechanism, as pain itself is not a physiological entity, but a multitude of varying neuroplastic changes being part of adaptive or maladaptive reactions.

THE EFFECTS OF ACUPUNCTURE ON PAIN

The effects of acupuncture on pain may be attributed to:

(1) peripheral effects (release of adenosine, NO, axonal and dorsal rot reflexes);
(2) spinal effects (modulation of sympathetic tone and motor reflexes);
(3) modulation of descending pain inhibitory and facilitatory systems;
(4) change in the functional connectivity of the brain, with activation or deactivation of:
  (a) limbic structures involved in stress/illness responses,
  (b) the HPA-axis, or
  (c) the prefrontal and frontal cortices;
(5) restoration of the default mode state;
(6) increase in parasympathetic activity;
(7) activation of the reward and mirror systems;
(8) modulation of the immune system;
(9) extinction of fear and anxiety induced behaviour; or
(10) expectation and attention.

Clinical trials suggest that variability in treatment outcome following acupuncture may also to a significant degree be attributed to the therapist. The importance of therapeutic alliance in predicting treatment success is well established. Also, acupuncture is part of a healing ritual allowing for a therapeutic alliance between the acupuncturist and the patient. Possibly this may be attributed to the ability to mediate empathy and/or consolation.

BACKGROUND

The human biological system has evolved over a very long period of time, yet remains adapted to a hunter-gatherer lifestyle where persistence in physical activity was of fundamental importance for survival. In modern society, psychosocial stress is high and motor activity frequently minimal, and the resulting emotional tension cannot be transformed into physical exercise in accordance with inherited biological needs. Instead, the stress-induced changes remain and can cause long-lasting disturbances in muscle tone and autonomous activity, resulting in various types of pain and functional diseases. A contributing factor to health disturbances is probably limited physical exercise with insufficient afferent input for an optimal performance. Changes in biological parameters occur as a result of somatic afferent stimulation whether from normal physical exercise, electrical stimulation of afferent nerve fibres or stimulation via acupuncture needles. The details of the underlying mechanisms are largely unknown, but most likely homeostatic and allostatic mechanisms are involved. The direction of change seems to be towards an optimal performance of different functions.

PAIN AND ACUPUNCTURE

In recent years, many publications have explored the effects of acupuncture in pain. 'Acupuncture' as a treatment encompasses much more than simply needling: it involves a complex interaction and context that may include empathy, touch, intention, expectation and conditioning. This is almost certainly why clinical research consistently demonstrates large effects from 'acupuncture' as a package of care, and small but statistically significant effects (Vickers *et al.*, 2012) of needling over "sham" techniques — that often involve needling as well — and as such may be considered a modality of sensory stimulation.[1]

Some patients may experience a reduction of their suffering which is paralleled by changes in biological parameters whereas others 'only' report a subjective relief i.e. the changes seen during and after a treatment are highly dependent on the subjective report of the patient and the pathophysiological pain mechanisms involved. This could account for some of the reasons why variable results of pain alleviation in response to acupuncture have been reported. Also, age and gender related variations in perceived pain have been discussed. Variability in outcome may also be attributed to

---

[1] Lewith and Cummings. Personal communication, 2012.

factors such as operationalisation of the outcome variable and the statistical method for evaluation. When pain is regarded as subjective, the produced data should be treated as ordinal. A rank-based method, taking the non-metric qualities of the ordinal data into account as well as the variability at the group and the individual level, may then be used. When using such an approach evaluating changes in electrical sensory thresholds and electrical pain thresholds after low-frequency electro-acupuncture separately (in men and women) it was found that outcomes were divergent between women and men, i.e. unchanged sensory threshold after acupuncture at the group level in women while changed in men. On the other hand the assessed pain threshold after acupuncture was changed towards higher levels in women and unchanged in men suggesting that there might be gender specific effects (Lund and Lundeberg, 2010). Likely there are many other causes of variability (including different aetiological factors) that have not yet been investigated and that are hidden within many of the statistical approaches.

Pain Classification

The paradigm of Traditional Chinese Medicine (TCM) with its balancing of energy may, in its way, explain diseases or disturbances, but it is from a Western perspective a philosophical rather than biological approach. In many of the original studies regarding acupuncture and pain the underlying mechanisms, e.g. pain relief, were often discussed relative to traditional TCM or to the location of the pain (for example low back pain, headache and knee pain) but surprisingly few studies have dealt with the effects of acupuncture in relation to the pathophysiological mechanisms involved.

In contrast to symptomatic and/or diagnosis-based pain treatments, mechanism-based treatments are more likely to succeed. Pain can be an adaptive sensation, an early warning to protect the body from tissue injury (nociceptive pain). By the introduction of hypersensitivity to normally innocuous stimuli, pain may also aid in repair after tissue damage (inflammatory pain). Pain can also be maladaptive, reflecting pathological function of the nervous system (neuropathic pain or dysfunctional/ long lasting pain).

Multiple molecular and cellular mechanisms operate alone and in combination within the peripheral and central nervous systems to produce the different forms of pain. Elucidation of these mechanisms (including for example; peripheral and central sensitization, neuroplasticity following nerve injury, contribution of the sympathetic nervous system and dysfunction of the pain modulatory systems (disinhibition and central facilitation) as well as cognitive and affective factors) is key to the development of acupuncture techniques that specifically target or modulates underlying causes rather than just symptoms.

It has been suggested that an evidence-based approach to pain management is not always possible or beneficial to the patient. In the face of inconclusive evidence, a theory-based approach may help determine if the therapeutic effect of a given sensory stimulation has the possibility of being a useful clinical tool in the context of treating a particular patient's mechanism of pain generation. Further studies on mechanism-based classification and such classification-based treatments are essential (Thomas and Lundeberg, 1996).

PHYSIOLOGICAL MECHANISMS OF ACUPUNCTURE

Overview

Effects of acupuncture therapy occur at multiple levels in the nervous system, both in the peripheral tissue, at segmental (spinal) and central levels (Stener-Victorin and Wu, 2010).

Peripheral mechanisms: Insertion and manual or electrical stimulation of needles in skin and muscle activates A-alpha, -beta, -delta and C-fibers. In particular, activation of A-delta and C-fibers may be essential for modulating pain and autonomic nervous system activity. Manual and electrical stimulation (electro-acupunture, EA) causes release of neuropeptides including calcitonin gene-related, peptide (CGRP) and vasoactive intestinal polypeptide (VIP) from peripheral nerve terminals and other vasodilatory mediators from the tissue around the needle (including adenosine and nitrous oxide, NO) into the area increasing blood flow. Interestingly, low-frequency (2 Hz pulse trains) EA also increase skeletal muscle glucose uptake. In insulin-resistant rats peripheral insulin sensitivity is improved by low-frequency EA for 4–5 weeks with three treatments per week and normalized by five treatments per week. Taken together, these finding suggest that local needling may improve nutritive blood flow and glucose uptake, factors that may be be impaired in ischemic and degenerative pain conditions.

Segmental mechanisms: Needle stimulation of muscles results in the activation of descending; nociceptive ('pain') and sympathetic inhibitory systems — terminating in the spinal cord — within the same segments. This is how acupuncture, by using so-called segmental acupuncture points, may alter organ function by modulating sympathetic efferent activity. Also, using points segmentally related to a specific organ may modulate parasympathetic activity. As discussed above many organ diseases, results in visceral pain may be attributed to stress and increased sympathetic tone. This is of interest since many stress related organ diseases has been shown to have an increased concentrations of nerve growth factor (NGF), a marker of sympathetic activity, within the organ. In the ovaries for example, segmental low frequency EA for 20 minutes resulted in increased ovarian blood flow and decreased sympathetic activity. Further evidence that low-frequency EA modulates ovarian sympathetic nerve activity comes from studies in experimentally induced ovarian dysfunction. Gene and protein expression of markers of sympathetic were normalized after four weeks of low-frequency EA. Also, in rats with experimentally induced ovarian dysfunction, ovarian morphology was improved by thrice weekly treatment for 4–5 weeks as seen by a higher proportion of healthy ovarian follicles than in untreated rats. When treatment was increased to five times per week, low-frequency EA normalised oestrus cyclicity. This suggests that there exists is clear dose-response relationship.

Central mechanisms: When acupuncture needles are inserted, signals are transferred from the periphery to the central nervous system (CNS). Since CNS regulates homeostasis, pituitary hormone release may be affected. Acupuncture also modulates immune, endocrine and metabolic function via the CNS. Many brain areas, especially the hypothalamus, are involved in the effect of acupuncture. Acupuncture-induced release of CNS neuromodulators (peptides and hormones) seems to be essential for inducing functional changes in organ systems. The central hypothalamic beta-endorphin system is likely a key mediator of changes in autonomic functions, such as effects on the vasomotor centre, which decreases sympathetic tone. The latter and is reflected by improved blood pressure regulation and decreased muscle sympathetic nerve activity. Both exercise and low-frequency EA increase hypothalamic beta-endorphin secretion and decrease blood pressure and sympathetic nerve activity following a treatment. Naloxone, a my-opioid receptor antagonist, reverses these effects. Interestingly, repeated low-frequency EA and/or physical exercise significantly decrease high sympathetic nerve activity for a sustained period of time. This suggest that acupuncture both have short- and long-term effects and that the long-term effects are not seen until a sufficient number of treatments have been carried, i.e. assessing the effects of acupuncture after one or a few treatments is not possible.

It is likely that some off the long-term effects of acupuncture may be attributed to changes in the expression and synthesis of hypothalamic beta-endorphin. Interestingly, growing evidence suggests that the opioid system is deregulated both centrally and peripherally in many stress related conditions. This suggestion is supported by experimental and clinical studies of polycystic ovary syndrome (PCOS) where it has been reported that the opioid system is deregulated both centrally and peripherally. Hypothalamic beta-endorphin interacts with the hypothalamic-pituitary-ovarian axis by exerting a tonic inhibitory effect on the gonadotropin-releasing hormone (GnRH) pulse generator. As has been demonstrated, acupuncture affect the hypothalamic-pituitary-ovarian axis by modulating central beta-endorphin production and secretion, thereby influencing the release of hypothalamic GnRH and pituitary secretion of other hormones including the gonadotropins. Furthermore, in rats with experimentally induced PCOS, five low-frequency EA treatments per week for 4–5 weeks restored hypothalamic androgen receptor and GnRH protein expression. These changes were paralleled by normalised expression and synthesis of hypothalamic beta-endorphin supporting a pivotal role of hypothalamus in the long-term effects of acupuncture.

POSSIBLE MECHANISMS IN THE ALLEVIATION OF PAIN FOLLOWING ACUPUNCTURE

Overview

Medical acupuncture is based on the activation of mechanoreceptors in the skin, muscle and connective tissue in tendons and muscles. Depending

on how the acupuncture treatment is performed, different types of mechanoreceptors are activated. A majority of the described acupuncture points
are found in muscle tissue. When an acupuncture needle is inserted into a
muscle and rotated muscle spindles are activated. The information from
the spindle is conveyed into the spinal cord through Ia afferent nerves
resulting in a reflex whereby the muscle fibers around the acupuncture
needle are contracted. Further manipulation of the needle results in the
activation of ergo-receptors in the muscle, pressure receptors that are
commonly activated by strong muscle contraction. The activation of the
ergo-receptors is perceived as a strong stimulus by the patient, the so-
called needle sensation or *de qi*. *De qi* is often reported as a dull, aching,
burning or stinging sensation. Afferent activity from the ergo-receptors is
transmitted to the spinal cord in thin myelinated Aδ-fibers. From the dorsal horn of the spinal cord the information is conveyed in the spinothalamic tract to the thalamus and further on into the CNS. On its way to the
CNS ascending nerve fibers also project to areas in the mesencephalon
(PAG, periaqueductal gray), and neurons in medulla oblongata (RVM,
rostroventral medulla). From RVM descending nerve pathways project to
the spinal cord pursuing a modulating effect on nociceptive transmission

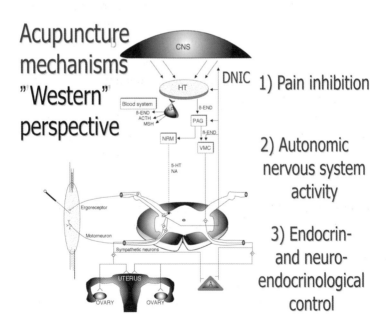

and sympathetic tone via the release of endogenous opioids (β-endorphins and enkephalins), monoamines (serotonin and nor epinephrine) and GABA (γ-amino-butyric acid) and glycine. Also, other 'pain' inhibitory systems, originating at the brain stem level exist. One of these is the DNIC mechanism (diffuse noxious inhibitory control system), which may be activated following intense and painful needle stimulation. Experimental studies suggest that this system has minor relevance in clinical practice.

From the thalamus, activity set up by the acupuncture needle is projected to limbic structures, somato-sensory cortex and frontal cortex. In the limbic structures needle stimulation results in a reduced activity (deactivation), which may result in a reduction of the affective component of a symptom. Also, the default mode is re-constituted. Deactivation of the limbic structures as well as a direct inflow from thalamus to hypothalamus will influence homeostasis and thereby influence hormonal release and autonomic regulation via the vasomotor centrum in the brain stem. Acupuncture also leads to deactivation of neuronal networks in the brain involved in avoidance behaviours and anxiety. Functional networks playing a role in reward and consolation are also activated.

A DEEPER LOOK INTO SOME OF THE POSSIBLE ANALGESIC EFFECTS OF ACUPUNCTURE

Peripheral Effects — Role of Adenosine

Acupuncture is commonly used to treat musculoskeletal pain and acupuncture points are often located in muscle tissue in close proximity to peripheral nerves thereby possibly intercepting nociceptive (pain) signals before they reach the spinal cord. Indeed it has been reported that adenosine, a neuromodulator with anti-nociceptive properties, is released locally during acupuncture in mice and that its anti-nociceptive actions required adenosine A1 receptor expression (A1R-dependent anti-nociception). Direct injection of an adenosine A1 receptor agonist replicated the analgesic effect of acupuncture. Inhibition of enzymes involved in adenosine degradation potentiated the acupuncture-elicited increase in adenosine, as well as its anti-nociceptive effect. The localised actions of acupuncture would hypothetically make acupuncture ideal for treating pain in specific regions of the body.

These findings triggered Hurt and Zylka (2012) to elucidate if the antinociception of adenosine/acupuncture could be transiently bosted with additional substrate (AMP), blocked with an A1 antagonist or an inhibitor of phospholipase C. They reported that injection of prostatic acid phosphatase (PAP), an ectonucleotidase that dephosphorylates extracellular AMP to adenosine, administered into the Weizhong acupuncture point at the popliteal fossa, had dose- and A1R-dependent antinociceptive effects in mice models of acute and chronic 'pain'. These inhibitory effects lasted up to six days following a single injection, much longer than the hour-long inhibition provided by acupuncture. Likely, PAP inhibits nociception via an A1R- and PLC-dependent mechanism in the periphery highlighting a role for this ectonucleotidase in peripheral pain mechanisms.

These novel findings show how deeper knowledge of acupuncture mechanisms may stimulate development of new treatments.

Given that a selective A1R antagonist blocked the antinociceptive effects of acupuncture and PAP, other compounds that block A1R, such as theophylline and caffeine (a non-selective A1 and A2 antagonist), could reduce the efficacy of acupuncture. Therefore, patients should probably eliminate xanthine-derived alkaloids (like caffeine) intake before treatment to maximise the analgesic effect of acupuncture. This suggestion is supported by a study showing that caffeine (but not placebo) at a dose equivalent to two to three cups of coffee can block the analgesic effects of transcutaneous electrical nerve stimulation (TENS).

The examples given above demonstrated how research into acupuncture mechanisms may result in new treatments, like local PAP administration, and how new findings may have direct impact on clinical practice i.e. that the analgesic effect of acupuncture partly may be attributed to a release of adenosine, a release possibly 'being at risk' by intake of coffee or soft drinks containing xanthine-derived alkaloids before treatment.

Spinal and Supraspinal Effects — Frequency Dependent Mechanisms

Just the fact that different modalities of acupuncture may have different effects suggests that the effects of acupuncture are related to the activation of various endogenous mechanisms (Han, 2011). If so selecting the appropriated modality is crucial when treating different pain conditions. The suggestion that different modalities of acupuncture activate different antinociceptive mechanisms is supported by studies showing that in rats with joint inflammation, there was an increased release of serotonin in the spinal cord during low (2 Hz), but not high frequency (100 Hz) EA. On the other hand, high-frequency, but not low-frequency EA reduced aspartate and glutamate release in the spinal cord. Also, in rats made tolerant to morphine, 2 Hz EA no longer had an anti-nociceptive effect, suggesting that low-frequency EA stimulates beta-endorphin release. If the two modes of stimulation indeed work through different mechanisms, they should not produce cross-tolerance with each other. This has been tested and the results show that prolonged stimulation with 2 Hz EA resulted in a gradual diminution of the analgesic effect, labelled as tolerance. Rats made tolerant to 2 Hz EA was fully responsive to 100 Hz, and vice versa, suggesting that they may be mediated by different receptors. This conclusion is also supported by a study in patients with dysmenorrhoea who reported that both high- and low-frequency TENS resulted in pain alleviation but only 2 Hz was reversed by the opioid antagonist naloxone. A modality specific effect on inflammation has also been reported. In a rat inflammatory model, 10 Hz EA, but not 100 Hz EA suppressed inflammation likely by activating the hypothalamus–pituitary–adrenal axis (HPA). Also, in a rat model of neuropathic 'pain' 2 Hz EA stimulation for 30 min suppressed cold hypersensitivity for more than 24 hours, whereas 100 Hz was without effect. Experimental studies in rats have explored the central pathways mediating low- and high-frequency EA analgesia. Two hertz EA sequentially activates the arcuate nucleus of the hypothalamus (beta-endorphinergic neurons), PAG, medulla (enkephalinergic neurons), and the dorsal horn to suppress nociceptive transmission whereas 100 Hz EA activate parabrachial nucleus-PAG-medulla-spinal dorsal horn to suppress nociceptive transmission. The '100 Hz pathway' involve the release of dynorphin.

Thus, the accumulating evidence suggests that 2 Hz and 100 Hz EA can be regarded as two distinct therapeutic entities. However, there is an individual variability in our ability to activated these systems as has been reported in patients with spinal cord injury pain subjected to different types of acupuncture, some preferring low frequency and others high frequency. This would suggest that the patients should be allowed to try different acupuncture stimulation techniques before selecting their mode of treatment.

Changes in Brain Activity Following Acupuncture

Neuroimaging has been used to both characterise evoked brain response to acupuncture needling, as well as assess longitudinal changes in brain activity in response to so-called acupuncture therapy 'translational' studies.

A recent meta-analysis (Huang *et al.*, 2012) investigating fMRI response to acupuncture needle stimulation found that brain response to acupuncture needle stimulation was characterised by a common pattern of activation and deactivation and different acupuncture points elicits overlapping response within multiple cortical, subcortical/limbic and brainstem areas. This would imply that acupuncture point specificity is not crucial from a brain perspective and that many of the effects of acupuncture in the brain are general. Areas with altered activity during and after activity include primary and secondary somatosensory cortices (SI, SII) and limbic brain regions (e.g. hypothalamus, amygdala, cingulate, hippocampus). The hippocampus plays and important role in learning and memory while the amygdala play a role in mood (affective processing). The limbic structures are directly connected to the brainstem as well as the hypothalamus. Neural network interaction between the amygdala/hippocampus and the hypothalamus affect arousal and the motivational state.

In general, many components of the limbic system are down regulated in response to acupuncture, specifically if the *de qi* sensation is induced. Furthermore, many acupuncture studies have demonstrated that acupuncture modulates the activity of anterior and posterior insula, and the prefrontal cortex (PFC). The prefrontal cortex, which has multiple connections with the limbic system, plays an important role in pain behaviour (avoidance reactions) as well as in expectancy. To elucidate the role of expectancy in acupuncture, comparisons to sham acupuncture have been made, and in a meta-analysis evidence of insula and cingulate activation and greater amygdala deactivation was found in response to real compared to sham acupuncture.

Other studies have found that resting brain connectivity (defined as ongoing neural and metabolic activity in the resting brain) is also modulated by acupuncture. Studies have reported that real, but not sham acupuncture, increased resting default mode network (DMN) connectivity immediately after needling (Dhond *et al.*, 2008). This result suggests that even after the needling procedure, there are sustained effects on brain activity. This is supported by studies showing decreased resting connectivity between the DMN and insula (areas involved in pain) over time following repeated acupuncture sessions.

To study the neurochemical processes involved in acupuncture PET have been used. Harris and coworkers (2009) investigated the action of acupuncture and sham acupuncture on mu-Opioid receptor (MOR) binding in fibromyalgia patients. They demonstrated that sham acupuncture caused a decrease in MOR binding ability whereas acupuncture increased receptor binding ability, within the same brain regions. In the acupuncture group, those individuals that displayed a greater increase in MOR binding were the also the patients that had improvements in clinical pain. Interestingly, while clinical pain was reduced to a similar extent in the acupuncture and the sham group, the MOR mechanisms were different. In another study Harris and collaborators used 1H-MRS to study glutamate and combined glutamate + glutamine (Glx) levels in patients with fibromyalgia following acupuncture (Harris *et al.*, 2008). They demonstrated that patients with greater reductions in glutamate and Glx displayed greater improvements in pain outcomes.

POSSIBLE CLINICAL IMPLICATIONS

Site of needle insertion: A combination of local needles in the area of pain, or within segmental receptive fields and distal (extrasegmental) needles in myotomes or sclerotomes to the origin of pain may be tried.

Intensity of stimulation: Pain decreased with either superficial needle insertion or deep mode acupuncture with *de qi*, but more patients responded to deep needling.

Duration of treatment: Thirty-minute treatment is effective. Longer treatment relieves similar numbers of patients, but greater numbers had increased pain.

Timing of intervention: Pre-emptive acupuncture analgesia may result in increased or decrease postoperative pain and analgesic consumption depending on time of intervention as has also been reported with opioids. On the other hand, treatment of chronic episodic dysmenorrhoea or migraine with acupuncture one week prior to menses/migraine reduced pain and analgesic consumption, or had no effect.

Mode of stimulation: Chronic nociceptive musculoskeletal pain is reduced by low-frequency electrical stimulation but also by manual acupuncture or high-frequency electrical stimulation. Periosteal stimulation has the greatest effect upon nociceptive visceral pain of dysmenorrhoea, although other modes of acupuncture and low-frequency TENS also reduced pain.

Aetiology of pain: In general patients with nociceptive or inflammatory/ischemic pain had a better effect of acupuncture as compared to patients with maladaptive pain (neuropathic or long-term pain).

SUMMARY

The term 'acupuncture' covers a diverse academic field that spans from ancient medical history to the most advanced contemporary neurophysiology. Practice ranges from simple techniques that can be taught to patients to more sophisticated invasive techniques that are the basis for much of the field of neuromodulation.

'Acupuncture' as a treatment for pain encompasses much more than simply needling: it involves a complex interaction and context that may include empathy, touch, intention, attention, expectation and conditioning. This is almost certainly why clinical research consistently demonstrates large effects from 'acupuncture' as package of care, and small (but statistically significant) effects of needling over sham techniques (that often involve needling as well). Simple techniques can be taught to most healthcare workers, and this can empower pain services in the remotest regions where more expensive medicines or even the simplest analgesics may not be accessible. By contrast, within the centre of modern healthcare, where there is access to the latest scanning technology, the use of the simple slim filiform needles can greatly enhance the assessment of pain by applying a mechanical stimulus in different tissue layers and recording the patient's perception and recognition of symptoms (as proposed by the inofficial

IASP SIG for Pain). Acupuncture has been demonstrated to be cost-effective as a treatment modality in its own right and as a complement to drugs and other physical interventions. It should be emphasised that acupuncture is a relatively safe treatment with few side effects and not associated with an 'environmental load' (drug residues in the nature).

REFERENCES

Dhond R, Yeh C, Park K, Kettner N, Napadow V. Acupuncture modulates resting state connectivity in default and sensorimotor brain networks. *Pain* 2008; **136**: 407–418.

Han J-S. Acupuncture analgesia: areas of consensus and controversy. *Pain* 2011; **152**(suppl 3): S41–S48.

Harris R, Sundgren P, Pang Y, Hsu M, Petrou M, Kim S, McLean S, Gracely R, Clauw D. Dynamic levels of glutamate within the insula are associated with improvements in multiple pain domains in fibromyalgia. *Arthritis Rheum* 2008; **58**: 903–907.

Harris R, Zubieta J, Scott D, Napadow V, Gracely R, Clauw D. Traditional Chinese acupuncture and placebo (sham) acupuncture are differentiated by their effects on mu-opioid receptors (MORs). *Neuroimage* 2009; **47**(3): 1077–1085.

Huang W, Pach D, Napadow V, Park K, Long X, *et al.* Characterizing acupuncture stimuli using brain imaging with fMRI — a systematic review and meta-analysis of the literature. *PLoS ONE* 2012; **7**(4): e32960.

Hurt J, Zylka M. PAPcupuncture has localized and long-lasting antinociceptive effects in mouse models of acute and chronic pain. *Mol. Pain* 2012; **8**: 28.

Lund I, Lundeberg T. On the threshold — evaluation of variability in effects of acupuncture in a gender perspective. *Chin Med.* 2010; **5**: 32–41.

Stener-Victorin E, Wu X. Effects and mechanisms of acupuncture in the reproductive system. *Auton Neurosci* 2010; **157**: 1–2, 46–51.

Thomas M, Lundeberg T. Does acupuncture work? *Pain Clin. Updates* 1996; **IV**: 1–11. http://www.iasppain.org/AM/AMTemplate.cfm?Section=Home, Home&CONTENTID=7614&TEMPLATE=/CM/ContentDisplay.cfm&SECTION=Home,Home

Vickers A, Cronin A, *et al.* Acupuncture for chronic pain: individual patient data meta-analysis. *Arch Intern Med.* 2012; **172**(19): 1444–1453.

CHAPTER 2

EXPLANATORY NATURE, MODELS, NEEDS AND REQUIREMENTS FOR TESTING THEM

Stephen Birch

University College of Health Sciences
Campus Kristiania, Oslo, Norway

Abstract

What are traditionally based systems of acupuncture, TBSAs? How are they different from other styles of acupuncture? What is the nature of knowledge and what the assumptions about the nature of things that underlie TBSAs? How is this thinking different from the nature of knowledge and assumptions about the nature of things that underlie modern scientific knowledge of the world? This briefly explores these issues in relation to the notion of the 'explanatory' models underlying TBSAs and biomedical knowledge of the body. It will examine the impact of these differences on how we develop testable 'explanatory models' of TBSAs and the likely requirements of such studies. These differences affect how we conceive of clinical testing of TBSAs, raising difficult questions about the viability of 'explanatory' trials of TBSAs. These differences also affect how we conceive of testing the 'mechanisms' of traditionally based systems of acupuncture. To date these issues have not been dealt with in clinical or physiological testing of TBSAs. The issues are compounded further by the fact that there are many different types of TBSAs with very different stimulation methods. This diversity challenges our assumptions about the nature of TBSAs and theories underlying them, making it difficult to make generalisations. The author believes that by looking behind this diversity and its ensuing complexity

S. Birch

it may be possible to grasp something about the nature of the theories underlying these systems. Alternative ways of conceiving of the concepts and purposes of TBSA systems of acupuncture are introduced, proposing that TBSA treatments may take advantage of low-level energy information regulation systems in the body.

INTRODUCTION

The term Traditional East Asian Medicine (TEAM) is defined here as those therapies of East Asian origin based on historical theories of the body in health and disease that are centred-upon the concept of *qi* [氣]. This includes traditionally based systems of acupuncture (TBSA) from Asia, and in recent decades the West. It also includes systems of herbal medicine (*zhongyao* [中藥]) practice such as the *bencao* [本草] traditions, Japanese *kampo* [漢方]. It also includes massage traditions such as *tuina* [推拿], *shiatsu* [指圧], and self-development traditions such as *taijiquan* [太極 拳], *qigong* [氣功] from Asia and in recent decades the West (see Fig. 1).

There have always been different TBSAs from the earliest to present times in the field of acupuncture.[13,19,22,91] Scholars tracing the development

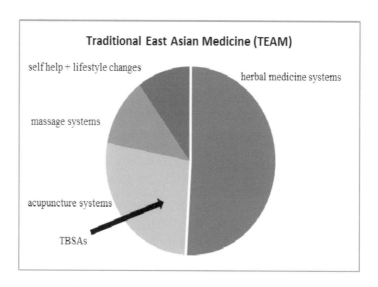

Fig. 1.   Traditional East Asian medical therapies.

of acupuncture from the period just before to the publication of the first acupuncture related texts of the *'Huangdi Neijing'*, [黃帝內經] the *'Suwen'* [素問] and *'Lingshu'* [靈樞] summarise the role of the acupuncture needle as a treatment instrument for regulating *qi*: "Needling regulates (tunes) the *qi* (*tiao qi* [調氣])" (Ref. 88, pp. 79, quoting chapter 75 of the *Lingshu*). Leading scholar Vivien Lo says of acupuncture "I differentiate 'acupuncture' from bloodletting and other minor surgery by the target of medical intervention. Acupuncture, as I define it, is the act of piercing the body with the intention of moving *qi* in the channels". (Ref. 63, pp. 29) But acupuncture has not always involved the insertion of acupuncture needles, from its first descriptions in the Lingshu, it has also involved use of 'needles' with rounded ends that were pressed or rubbed on the surface of the body as non-insertion forms of acupuncture (Ref. 21, pp. 45–54; Ref. 64, pp. 102–103), techniques which are still in use today.[21,35,95] Needling has always been at different depths, including very shallow needling.[27] Needling as a treatment method was introduced after the use of moxa cauterization had already been described,[63,64,104] hence the frequent use of the term [鍼灸] *'zhenjiu'* (Japanese 'shinkyu') 'acumoxa therapy' to refer to acupuncture. Treatment with needles or moxa is directed to the acupuncture points or *'xue'* [穴], the most important of which are located along the twelve *jingmai* [經脈] or channels. The twelve jingmai are a development from an earlier primitive physiological concept, the *'mai'* [脈], first described in texts found in the *Zhanjiashan*.

[張家山] (circa 196–186 BCE) and the *Mawangdui* [馬王堆] (circa 168 BCE) archaeological sites [32, 39]. The term *'jing'* [經] can be understood in a number of ways, but scholars of the period usually understand it as implying order or regularity [e.g. Ref. 96], so that the term *jingmai* is about ordering the physiology (*mai*) of the body. Thus the principle purpose of a system of acupuncture following traditional theories of acupuncture (TBSAs) is to apply needling techniques in order to restore order to the *qi*, to help regulate the *qi*. This is a core idea underlying TBSAs, but one that has found many means of expression, with varying degrees of emphasis and different understanding of how to do this. To understand this more I turn to an examination of the theories of TBSAs, in particular their role as 'explanatory models'.

In the modern period acupuncture has been shown to be a 'complex intervention' especially traditionally based systems of acupuncture.[5,68,80,81,89,91] Complex interventions need to be carefully defined and often have much more complex mechanisms of action and inter-action.[29,72]

EXPLANATORY MODELS

Today, if we talk about explanatory models of a therapy we are referring to the mechanisms and physiological pathways through which that therapy is thought to act. Therapy x acts on physiological pathway y to trigger change z which reduces the symptom. In this model there is a chain of causal events (x-y-z) between the therapy and the change of symptom. In clinical research the explanatory trial is "aimed at confirming a physiological hypothesis, precisely specified as a causal relationship between administration of an intervention and some physiological outcome".[102]

Stephen Hawking, arguably the world's greatest scientist recently wrote about models: "Whenever we develop a model of the world and find it to be successful, we tend to attribute to the model the quality of reality or absolute truth. But ... the same physical situation can be modelled in different ways, each employing different fundamental elements and concepts. It might be that to describe the universe we have to employ different theories in different situations. Each theory may have its own version of reality, but according to model-dependent realism, that diversity is acceptable, and none of the versions can be said to be more real than any other".[40] Such a conclusion from one of the world's leading scientists makes us raise questions about simple ideas such as the 'explanatory model' and assumptions and conclusions we might draw from it.

In acupuncture we find three kinds of 'explanatory' models, the first a mechanistic one, the second proposed on the basis of known physiology and the third based on traditional qi-based descriptions of the body. The first arises out of research on a particular clinical outcome. For example if acupuncture is said to reduce pain, what mechanisms must or could be involved for the therapy to be able to reduce the pain? The hypothesised mechanism that reduces the pain is worked out with evidence showing a relationship between the input (acupuncture) and the measured output (release of endorphins resulting in pain reduction). When these physiological models are demonstrated through careful research, then an explanatory model of acupuncture in the treatment of pain is thought to be confirmed.[25,83] Hammerschlag and colleagues pointed out that this line of evidence does not actually expose the mechanisms involved rather it establishes correlation between the input of acupuncture and the measured output.[37, 38] The actual mechanisms of acupuncture remain unclear.[37,38] But additionally this line of reasoning provides evidence only for a limited use of acupuncture, e.g. pain reduction, and does not cover the broader use of acupuncture for conditions unaffected by the specific physiological pathway. It is dubious whether such models are 'explanatory models' of acupuncture, though they might eventually be valid as explanations for some of the effects of acupuncture.

The second explanatory model utilises known physiological entities and their pathways of action. This kind of explanatory model proposes that acupuncture works through those entities, for example, that acupuncture points are trigger points and that acupuncture works via the same mechanisms that trigger points work. This kind of model is developed by replacing the original concepts of acupuncture with more plausible sounding established biomedical concepts (replacement models). In the case of the proposed model that acupuncture is really dry needling of trigger points, certain challenges remain. For example, the claim that acupuncture points and trigger points are identical remains problematic,[14,15] there are on-going problems with the identification of trigger points,[65] trigger point needling has yet to demonstrate efficacy beyond placebo[31,50] while acupuncture has demonstrated efficacy beyond placebo in a number of medical conditions (e.g. Ref. 44, 58 and 60). In the case of trigger points as an explanatory model of acupuncture, many unresolved problems exist. This second kind of explanatory model the 'replacement' models of acupuncture, point to experimental evidence, without mapping the practice of acupuncture to those models and often little clinical trial evidence exists of the efficacy of those models of treatment. It is dubious whether these are really 'explanatory models' of acupuncture, and until the evidence is sufficient, judgement about their validity should be suspended.

The third type of explanatory model developed as acupuncture began developing in the period 150–100 BCE and is used by TBSAs. They make reference to concepts such as *qi* [氣], *jingmai* [經脈] (meridians), *xue* [穴]

(acu-holes), needling to regulate *qi* [調氣], *xu-shi* [虛實] (weakness-excess), *bu-xie* [補寫], (strengthen-drain), and so on. Many different models of acupuncture practice evolved over this more than two thousand year history, each selecting from and applying different aspects of the traditional ideas based on individual practitioner education, preferences, cultural background and clinical experiences.[19,22,67,90,91] The fact that such diversity exists and that different models of practice appear to have contradictory theories suggests that the theoretical models of practice may be problematic as 'explanatory' models in the sense defined above. To understand this I explore the kind of thinking and underlying world view assumptions that were made as these traditional theories and ideas developed. For, as we will see, it does not seem likely that the traditional ideas were intended to be nor could they function as 'explanatory models' that establish "a causal relationship between administration of an intervention and some physiological outcome." The theories of TBSAs seem to function differently.

TEAM THEORIES

There are profound differences in the ways of thinking and assumptions about the nature of the world in TEAM and modern scientific descriptions of the body [22]. Appendix 1 describes the core differences, here I summarise them very briefly. The assumptions about the nature of the world that lie at the heart of TEAM practices from the time of their inception (200–100 BCE) until now are largely characterised by the following features: Rather than seek the nature of things through breaking them down to smaller and smaller units (reductionist approach) there has been a tendency in TEAM to see things as parts of irreducible wholes, focusing especially on their relationships and mutual actions (syncretic thinking) (not to be confused with 'holism' — see Appendix 1). In TEAM thinking there is a virtual absence of seeking objective descriptions of the world and a virtual absence of the 'either-or' thinking that lies at the heart of the scientific method. Knowledge was more of the nature of 'skill-knowledge' (action oriented, describing things in ways that allowed actions to address problems in the world) rather than the 'representational knowledge' of modern science.[97]

In systems of practice where knowledge is not of objective causally related phenomena, rather of action oriented theories that help address problems in the world, what can we say about those theories? Traditional theories and models of the world including the medical theories of TEAM such as the *qi* and *jingmai*, play a different role than modern scientific theories. A very reasonable explanation of the role of theory in TEAM and subsequently TBSAs is that it refers to functional concepts that are primarily about guiding clinical judgments in order to select what the practitioner considers to be an optimal treatment within the system of practice he uses (Ref. 19, pp. 222; Ref. 78). Of course the patterns of diagnosis used within different systems of TEAM practice (e.g. Refs. 94, 110) can be seen as referring to phenomena that are associated with the problems of the patient but such association cannot be taken as 'causally related' until studies have been done that establish them to be causal relationships.

THE CHALLENGES OF TBSA EXPLANATORY MODELS

Now that the basic issues have been outlined, problems in the conceptualisation and testing of explanatory models of TBSAs can be examined. Three main areas will be discussed: (1) the explanatory RCT, (2) basic science of TBSAs, and (3) the need for a broader view of TBSAs.

The Explanatory RCT

Since an explanatory RCT is "aimed at confirming a physiological hypothesis, precisely specified as a causal relationship between administration of an intervention and some physiological outcome",[102] we can see immediate problems for explanatory trials of TBSAs. Despite what proponents of TBSAs might say, until studies have been conducted establishing objective causal relationships between the TBSA theories and (some) physiological outcome(s), the theories of each TBSA cannot be 'explanatory' in the sense defined here. Thus 'explanatory' trials of TBSAs are problematic. Arguments have recently been published drawing similar conclusions.[56] Not only are the 'mechanisms' of acupuncture unclear in TBSAs since the theories could not describe the mechanisms of treatment, but the mechanisms of acupuncture (explanatory model one above) remain unclear.[37,38] There remains the further problem that if the mechanisms are unclear, then what constitutes a viable placebo control remains unclear.[56] Attempts to conduct 'explanatory trials' of acupuncture have focussed on testing only one or two key variables: the location of needling, or the type of needling.[20,109] While these are important features of acupuncture practice, they do not constitute an explanatory model since we do not have definitive answers yet about the physiological basis of 'acupoints' or the different needling techniques. Further, evidence has shown that TBSAs are complex interventions[4,5,56,68,80,81,89,91] and reducing the theories of these to two variables such as point location and needling technique does not reflect TBSA practice nor can it tell us about the explanatory models of TBSAs. I do not dwell on these difficult issues further as these are not the main theme of the current paper, but it seems unlikely at present that clinical trials of a TBSA can test the mechanisms of the treatment and that 'explanatory' RCTs of TBSAs may not be possible as a test of the theories or mechanisms of TBSAs.

Basic Science of TBSAs

What steps are needed in order to investigate TBSA concepts such as '*qi*' or '*jingmai*' so that the hypothesis that they may have an objective basis can be tested and if so, what their physiological bases might be? Put another way, how do we ensure the validity of any claims to have established the objective existence of or physiological basis of these concepts and theories? This is a theme I have addressed in a separate paper,[18] so here I summarise the core ideas. A number of studies have been done and various claims made regarding the nature of concepts such as *qi*, the acupoints, the *jingmai*/channels, *deqi*, etc. However, no studies to date have addressed the issue that the concepts that were investigated are, by nature, functional concepts that guide clinical practice, were not described as having an objective nature and if observed have always been observed by the naked senses. Birch and Bovey argue that any measurements must be matched to reliable observations associated with the entity investigated and that as functional concepts their behaviour must also be assessed.[18] For example, after making observations of the entity, make measurements using the selected technology, then apply treatment to create a change in that entity, confirm those changes through reliable observation, then repeat the measurement to see if changes can be detected. This is based on the idea that measurable changes should match predicted changes based on theories of the entity. These are two fundamental steps that have been missing in research to date. Additionally, since there are important variations within the TBSA literature so that concepts from that literature are often described in different ways, significant work needs first to be done to establish reasonably agreed upon models of the entity to be investigated. Often this step is also poorly attended by researchers as it requires the work of historians, linguists, anthropologists who do not usually work with laboratory researchers.[18] Once agreed upon models are developed it may also be necessary to tighten up the hypotheses using mathematical modelling approaches so that sufficiently precise hypotheses can be generated.[18] Another area where insufficient attention has been given is in the choice of measurement technologies, there is rarely sufficient evidence given and arguments provided to justify the choice of those technologies. Birch and Bovey summarise this in an iterative nine-step process.[18]

The Need for a Broader View of TBSAs

How are we to understand the theoretical concepts of TBSAs? In principle they are based on concepts embedded in different perspectives of the nature of the world than many concepts in biology and medicine.[34] Ignoring these perspectives runs the risk of reducing the validity of any studies and their findings. Thus it is helpful to think about how to model these theories in ways that respects the underlying theories, a step mentioned by researchers grappling with the investigation of therapies as a whole system or as a complex intervention.[29,108] We may also have to accept quite different descriptions as valid even though they may appear contradictory.[40] Since the theories refer to ideas that are functional entities rather than obviously anatomical entities then it might be useful to consider these ideas as describing more subtle phenomena that function not as the physiological processes themselves (which have been well defined in modern biological terms already) but rather as systems that influence or even help regulate physiological systems. Yoshio Manaka developed a line of reasoning that hints at this. He studied acupuncture widely, the variety of historical and modern ideas and methods that can be found.[70] In his efforts to investigate TEAM based practices, he was looking for a practical solution to the following problem: If the traditional theories (*jingmai, qi*, yin-yang, etc.) are 'real' how can they be investigated when accessed by so many different styles and levels of stimulation — TCM needling — simple non-stimulatory needling — Japanese Meridian Therapy inserted needling — various non-penetrating needling? He realised that this is like looking for the lowest common denominator in a sequence of numbers such as: $2 - 8 - 30 - 68 - 188 - 368$. The only thing they have in common is the number 1 or 2. If different styles of acupuncture administer different levels of stimulation intensity and each claims to be accessing the same systems (*qi, jingmai*, etc.) then it can only be by the lowest intensity stimulus that they can do this, as this is the only thing they all have in common. Thus, if the TEAM concepts of *qi, jingmai*, etc. are anything more than 'software'.[70] or rules for applying treatment,[19] they must operate at very low energy levels. Further if the goal of acupuncture is to 'regulate the *qi*' [調氣] (Lingshu chapter 75 is explicit about this, Ref. 88, pp. 79) then perhaps these low-energy level phenomena are rather about regulation of the body. He then proceeded through a series of investigations to explore the nature of qi, the jingmai, their acupoints and proposed the model of 'acupuncture as intervention in the biological information system'.[69] While his experimental evidence is weak due to flaws in the studies his underlying ideas are worth further consideration. He proposed that perhaps modelling acupuncture in the framework of for example systems theory, information theory, complexity theory may be helpful as they allow perspectives of the body that don't appear to violate underlying TEAM assumptions about the nature of the world and the body's place in it.[70]

To make this clearer let's look briefly at a series of different types of needling: non-penetrating needling[35]/very lightly inserted needling (0.5–1.0 mm) with no sensation[94,95]/slightly more deeply inserted needling (2–5mm) with no sensation[21,70]/deeper insertion intramuscularly (5–20+mm) with no sensation[21]/deeper insertion needling (5–20+mm) with sensations — called *deqi* [得 氣] in many forms of acupuncture today.[85] All levels of needling activate 'bio-information'. The term 'bio-information' as used here refers to all biological structures and their functional systems, it also refers to the multiple control and regulatory systems that operate within and between biological organisms, it also refers to the flow of information from outside the body into the body and its biological responses/adaptations. A good general model for this can be found in the book '*Anti-chance*' by Schoffeniels,[92] the conceptual basis of this model of bio-information is found in detail in '*The Second Medical Revolution*' by Foss and Rothenberg[34] as well as more recently by Bischof[23] and Rein.[87]

As the needling is applied at different depths with different levels of stimulus, it is not difficult to imagine that different physiological systems are being accessed.

5- At the deeper anatomical level with sensory stimulation sensations, various mechanisms within the CNS and endocrine systems can become activated.

4- At the deeper anatomical level with minimal or no sensory stimulation, these same mechanisms may be activated, but likely to a much lesser degree if at all, instead the local tissues (muscular, connective tissue, vascular, local nerves) will be activated in varying degrees and amounts.

3- At the more shallow insertion levels with no sensory stimulation, if the needling is not intramuscular, the muscle tissues will not be involved in responses rather local subcutaneous tissue structures (vascular, connective tissue, etc.) will be activated.

2- With very shallow insertion, the skin and subcutaneous tissues will be the only systems activated, including surface sensory nerves, perhaps pressure receptors, current of injury response from the penetration of and small damage to the skin, etc.

1- With non-inserted needling, few of the mechanisms described above will be activated and responses will be due to other input.

With level five stimulation methods it is possible to see responses from all levels 1–5. With level four stimulation it is possible to see responses from all levels 1–4, and so on for the other levels. All inputs (stimulation levels) are a form of bio-information flow and all responses are a form of bio-information flow. This conceptual framework provides a 'paradigm' neutral and 'style of practice' neutral language that permits all systems and ideas to co-exist.

What might the information flows from each level involve? The skin contains 'polymodal receptors' that are likely to play a role in this information processing [52] and which will be present regardless of the level of stimulation. Touch is involved in all levels and can trigger different effects.[33,57,71] Gentle needling techniques can increase parasympathic tone.[76] Evidence is gradually accumulating that healing intention can have positive physiological effects[86] which could occur regardless of needling style. Various studies have documented that acupuncture points and the acupuncture channels have electromagnetic properties. In particular there is a body of research documenting that acupuncture points have low electrical resistance or higher conductance than surrounding skin and some has found that the acupuncture channels also have lower electrical resistance or higher conductivity.[2,9,10,73,74,93,99,100,111] Various theories exist about the electrical properties, characteristics and their functions.[12,79] The most common is that organisms use low-level energy signals as a mechanism for transmitting information within the body and as a mechanism for receiving and processing information from the environment. Various authors have speculated on the essential nature of these electro-magnetic fields and functions.[3,26,79] Others have drawn correlations between the electrical properties of the acupuncture systems (points and channels) and various bio-electrical systems such as the 'primitive DC electrical' system involved in growth and repair,[9,10] bio-informational signaling systems,[62] in particular the X-signal system,[70] point singularity theory,[93] bio-coherence models,[42,43] signal transmission and reception.[101] In most of these models, the EM signals communicate information that helps change physiological behavior and are often regulatory in nature.

Boon *et al.* in a review of different whole systems and complex systems research approaches stated "both the human body and systems of healthcare have to be seen as complex, self-organizing systems that create new, emerging properties through the interplay of their component elements".[24] Something like this seems to be appropriate to characterise TBSAs. In the TBSA, where the theories of action are not clear, there appears to be a complex model of potential action which depends in part on the nature of the treatment technique applied, in part on the selected locations for application of those techniques and various other factors guided by the TBSA theories that involve how the patient is engaged by the therapist, how the practitioner and patient interact,[108] how practitioner perceptions influence and thus modify the application of the treatment, etc. These different factors participate in interactive processes in the treatment. Systems and information theory modelling appear to be helpful tools for capturing and modelling this. Likewise, complexity theory and the development of order out of disorder (chaos theory) also appear to be helpful ways of modelling these processes. Most likely acupuncture treatment involves multiple levels of biological actions including established biological pathways and potentially other emerging pathways related to EM signals in the body. How TBSAs engage these and how well TBSA theories approximate, match, describe these or have nothing to do with them remain unclear. As Manaka described, the factors involved are likely to be very subtle or operate at very low energy levels, which, without the right technology, can be very difficult to detect and map. Demonstrating measurable phenomena that match the theories is the first order of business. Reproducing these results and calibrating them to TBSA theories and established physiological mechanisms or models will take time. If such efforts are successful, then will it be possible to design studies to test the explanatory models of TBSAs.

CONCLUSIONS

The theories underlying the practice of TBSAs serve primarily as guides on how to assess, diagnose and treat patients. They are not by nature, 'explanatory models' in the sense that biomedicine uses this term, describing cause and effect relationships between identified 'diagnoses' and disease or symptoms or between selected treatments and change of those symptoms or diseases. Explanatory models of TBSAs thus remain unclear. Appropriate models, hypotheses and evidence have yet to be developed. A number of steps are needed to do this with little work done so far in this direction. This paper has reviewed this topic, identified problems in both clinical and basic science research on TBSAs in relation to testing their explanatory models and suggested models and ways of thinking that may help future research in this area.

APPENDIX 1

A number of authors have written about the philosophical differences between Western, scientifically influenced world views and their assumptions and more traditional East Asian world views and assumptions (e.g. Refs. 36, 55, 84). Paul Unschuld captured some of these issues especially as they pertain to understanding the medical literatures;[103,105,106] Birch has recapitulated some of them.[11,13,19,22] While there is a tendency to try to argue on the basis of 'paradigmatic' differences between East and West [e.g. 11] following the arguments of Kuhn,[54] there are counter-arguments about the inadequacy of that approach.[53,90,104] Unschuld argues that 'Thomas Kuhn's notions of 'scientific revolution' and 'periods of normal science' are hardly applicable to Chinese history of science' (Ref. 104, pp. 6, 7). Scheid and others argue further that Pickering's 'mangle of practice' model[82] is more suitable to understand how East and West differences can be examined.[53,90] We will thus not engage in arguments or discussions further about paradigmatic differences, instead focusing here on a number of important philosophical differences. For more detailed discussions of the following, see the authors cited above and also Birch, and Bovey.[18]

There has been a virtual lack of 'objectivity' in traditional East Asian thinking. The theory of objectivity proposes that the person observing and describing the world is able to separate himself from it and describe it independent of himself as observer.[34] This approach is based on the assumptions that the person observing does not influence what is observed and that they are able to separate themselves from their observations. The objective world is described once individual experiences of the world are superceded. This trend did not happen in East Asia (Ref. 36, pp. 15; Ref. 61, pp. 192, 193) until the adoption of Western ways of thinking in recent centuries.[19,22] Instead, the observer was always placed at the centre of observations and there was not a tendency to try to describe things objectively. The individual was conceived as part of a larger whole and thus individual experiences of the world could not be separated from the world that is experienced. On this issue Sivin and Lloyd said "objectivity did not become an issue" (Ref. 61, pp. 192) and "Scientific pursuits in China thus did not aim at stepwise approximations to an objective reality but at recovery of what the archaic sages already knew" (Ref. 61, pp. 193).

There has been a virtual lack in traditional East Asian thinking of the 'either-or' thinking that is a hallmark of the scientific approach. In the either-or assumptive model, one cannot accept the validity of competing ideas; if one idea is considered right a contradictory one must be wrong. The scientific method for establishing 'truth' is a clear example of the either-or approach. Scientific truth is developed using methods that assume this to be axiomatic. While it has dominated modern Western scientific thinking, its virtual absence in ancient Asian philosophies is often overlooked. Evidence from the medical field clearly demonstrates a corpus of traditional literature that is full of contradictory ideas, even within the same texts, the absence of 'either-or' thinking is normal (Ref. 96, pp. 81). TEAM was fundamentally syncretistic, it has always employed a strategy of merging disparate ways of thinking and acting. This was not a problem for early authors since they did not assume that if one approach was right the other had to be wrong. Rather, ideas and assumptions of all kinds coexist at many different 'levels' of interpretation with no attempt or indeed any reason to derive an absolute truth. Of this Unschuld has written "The unique feature of the Chinese situation — and this should receive more attention from historians and philosophers of science — is the continuous tendency towards a syncretism of all ideas that exist (within accepted limits). Somehow a way was always found in China to reconcile opposing views and to build bridges" (Ref. 103, pp. 57).

There is a potential inapplicability of reductionist thinking to the primarily syncretistic thinking of traditional East Asian thinking. The reductionist approach is based on the assumptions that any whole system properties of a thing are nothing more than the simple sum of the parts of that thing and that the reduction of the thing to its component parts does not diminish the thing or our understanding of the thing itself. The opposite tendency has dominated in East Asian thinking due largely to the tendency to see things as part of an inseparable whole.[75] While this model of holism has not been universal in pre-medical and medical traditions in East Asia[105,106] it has certainly played very significant roles in how the mind and body were viewed and how they are seen in relation to the world and others. Ames and Hall in a discussion of the "most crucial contribution of Chinese culture broadly" cite Tang Junyi saying it is "...the spirit of the symbiosis and mutuality between particular and totality. In terms of our understanding this means an unwillingness to isolate the particular from the totality, and in terms of feeling, it means the commitment of the particular to do its best to realize the totality" (Ref. 6, pp. 11). Reductionism is rather an antithesis to this basic approach.

There has been a virtual lack of mind-body dualism in traditional East Asian thinking. In the 1600s the philosopher-mathematician Rene Descartes proposed that it is possible to view the mind and body separately with his famous '*cogito ergo sum*', 'I think therefore I am', creating the movement known as Descartian dualism.[34] This dualism did not start with Descartes, it had its origins with the ancient Greeks, further ramified by Christian theologians to become "one of the most influential problematics of modern philosophy" (Ref. 36, pp. 29) following Descartes. This has been very influential in Western thinking since he first proposed it with a strong trend in the Western view and in science to see the mind and body as separate, creating a kind of dualism. This has become an embedded part of the Western world view that is difficult to dislodge despite growing evidence in science that it is invalid.[34] In contrast to this, the ancient Chinese and TEAM perspective sees the mind and body as being completely inseparable: "the Chinese in contrast, accepted that the mind was part of the body, more refined and essentialized but of the same substance" (Ref. 59, pp. 20). While there have been occasional references that discussed mind and body as separate in the pre-medical (Ref. 30, pp. 152) and early TEAM literature (Ref. 28, pp. 165) and other discussions that seem to imply a similarity to the duality found in the West (Ref. 55, pp. 180), the bulk of the pre-medical and medical literature discusses them as inseparable.[3,6,30,45,59,84,107] We can thus reasonably take the continuity or inseparability of mind and body as typically but not exclusively representative of the early Chinese and TEAM traditions. Both are seen as different manifestations of *qi*.

Hypothesis testing in scientific studies. An important aspect of all hypothesis testing approaches relates to the underlying methodology that has to be used: in all hypothesis testing experiments, one never proves anything, one can only ever disprove competing, alternate or opposite hypotheses. Hence in all hypothesis testing studies the 'null hypothesis' (the opposite to the hypothesis) is tested. When it is proven to be wrong, it is assumed that the hypothesis was correct. But a fundamental limitation of this method is that it is entirely dependent on the starting assumptions and theories of the researchers (Ref. 22, pp. 30–31). In order to properly investigate TEAM concepts and methods it is necessary to have a detailed knowledge of the theories and methods of TEAM to ensure that valid and relevant ideas or methods are being investigated. Kim showed how a study of acupuncture began with a naive understanding and ultimately investigated models incapable of testing theories or concepts in acupuncture.[53] Accidentally or inadvertently, substituting biomedical ideas or models into studies that attempt to test TEAM will be problematic.

Taking the philosophical issues of the lack of objectivity and the lack of the 'either-or' assumption in traditional East Asian thinking, we are confronted with the question: 'What role does theory play in such a world view?' The philosophical argument regarding this perspective is that knowledge in ancient Chinese thinking was more 'skill-knowledge' rather than 'representational knowledge' (Ref. 97, pp. 4) or 'how-priority' knowledge rather than 'what-priority' knowledge (Ref. 36, pp. 149, 150). Hall and Ames state it clearly in different ways: "'Knowing,' then in classical China is not a knowing what that provides some understanding of the environment conditions of the natural world, but is rather a knowing how to be adept in relationships, and how in optimizing the possibilities that these relations provide, to develop trust in their viability" (Ref. 36, pp. 150). Kuriyama shows that in classical Chinese thinking "asking 'what' was inseparable from asking 'how'" (Ref. 55, pp. 96). The Western model of 'practice-knowledge' that seems to approximate this and which is commonly referenced is Polyani's 'tacit knowing' (Ref. 97, pp. 4). Slingerland explains it thus: "For the early Chinese thinkers ... the culmination of knowledge is understood not in terms of a grasp of abstract principles but rather as an ability to move through the world and human society in a manner that is completely spontaneous and yet still fully in harmony with the normative order of the natural and human worlds — the *Dao* or 'way'" (Ref. 97, pp. 4). We can thus see that there are important differences of world view between the ways that TEAM thinkers conceived of the world, the body, disease and treatment compared to modern scientifically influenced world views and their subsequent methods of investigation and practice. If we are to investigate TEAM theories, methods and practices we must be mindful of these differences and seek out approaches that do not ignore or bypass important features of the methods we attempt to investigate.

REFERENCES

1. Acupuncture. *NIH Consensus Statement* 1997; **15**(5): 1–34.
2. Ahn AC, Colbert AP, Anderson BJ, Martinsen OG, Hammerschlag R, Cina S, Wayne PM, Langevin HM. Electrical properties of acupuncture points and meridians: a systematic review. *Bioelectromagnetics* 2008; **29**(4): 245–256.
3. Allan S. *The Way of Water and Sprouts of Virtue*. Albany: State University of New York, 1997.
4. Alraek T, Birch S. Acupuncture research strategies — a commentary on the Society for Acupuncture Research white paper. *Forsch Komplementmed* 2012; **19**: 43–48, DOI: 10.1159/000336801.
5. Alraek T, Malterud K: Acupuncture for menopausal hot flashes: a qualitative study about patient experiences. *J Altern Complem Med* 2009; 15: 153–158.
6. Ames RT, Hall DL. *A Philosophical Translation: Dao De Jing — Making This Life Significant*. New York: Ballantine Books, 2003.
7. Anderson BJ. Integrating science and religion — implications for the scientific understanding of Chinese medicine Part I: an essay review of the marriage of sense and soul: Integrating science and religion by Ken Wilber. *Clin Acup Orient Med* 2002; **3**(1): 51–58.
8. Anderson BJ. Integrating science and religion — implications for the scientific understanding of Chinese medicine Part II: using Ken Wilber's integral vision as a basis for the integration of Chinese medicine and Western science. *Clin Acup Orient Med* 2003; **4**(1): 1–10.
9. Becker RO, Marino AA. *Electromagnetism and Life*. Albany: State University of New York Press, 1982.
10. Becker RO, Selden G. *The Body Electric*. New York: William Morrow, 1985.

11. Birch S. Introduction. In: Manaka Y, Itaya K, Birch S eds. *Chasing the Dragon's Tail.* Brookline: Paradigm Publications, 1995a: pp. 9–27.

12. Birch S. Further thoughts about the possible nature of the X-signals. In: Manaka Y, Itaya K, Birch S eds. *Chasing the Dragon's Tail.* Brookline: Paradigm Publications, 1995b: pp. 413–423.

13. Birch S. Diversity and acupuncture: Acupuncture is not a coherent or historically stable tradition. In: Vickers AJ. ed. *Examining Complementary Medicine: The Sceptical Holist.* Cheltenham: Stanley Thomas, 1998: pp. 45–63.

14. Birch S. Trigger point — acupuncture point correlations revisited. *J Alt Complem Med* 2003; **9**(1): 91–103.

15. Birch S. Trigger points should not be confused with acupoints. *J Alt Complem Med* 2008; **14**(10): 1184–1185.

16. Birch S. Filling the whole in acupuncture. Part 1: What are we doing in the supplementation needle technique? *EJOM*, 2009; **6**(2): 25–35 (part 1); 2009; **6**(3): 18–27 (part 2).

17. Birch S. Sham acupuncture is not a placebo treatment — implications and problems in research. *JAM* (in press).

18. Birch S, Bovey M. Scientific investigation of concepts based in traditional East Asian Medicine: Challenges to cross-paradigm research (in preparation).

19. Birch S, Felt R. *Understanding Acupuncture.* Edinburgh: Churchill Livingstone, 1999.

20. Birch S, Hammerschlag R, Trinh K, Zaslawski C. The non-specific effects of acupuncture treatment: When and how to control for them. *Clin Acupunct Orient Med* 2002; **3**: 20–25.

21. Birch S, Ida J. *Japanese Acupuncture: A Clinical Guide.* Brookline: Paradigm Publications, 1998.

22. Birch S, Lewith G. Acupuncture research, the story so far. In: MacPherson H, Hammerschlag R, Lewith G, Schnyer R eds. *Acupuncture Research: Strategies for Building an Evidence Base.* London: Elsevier, 2007: pp. 15–35.

23. Bischof M. Field concepts and the emergence of a holistic biophysics. In: Beloussov LV, Popp FA, Voeikov VL, Van Wijk R eds. *Biophotonics and Coherent Systems.* Moscow: Moscow University Press; 2000: pp. 1–25.

24. Boon H, MacPherson H, Fleishman S, Grimsgaard S, Koithan M, Norheim AJ, Walach H. Evaluating complex healthcare systems: a critique of four approaches. *eCAM* 2007; **4**(3): 279–285. doi:10.1093/ecam/nel079

25. Bowsher D. Mechanisms of acupuncture. In: Filshie J White A eds. *Medical Acupuncture*. Edinburgh: Churchill Livingstone, 1998: pp. 69–83.

26. Burr HS. *The Fields of Life*. New York: Ballantine Books, 1972.

27. Chace C. On greeting a friend, an approach to needle technique. *Lantern* 2006; **3**(3): 4–7.

28. Chiu ML. Mind, body, and illness in a Chinese medical tradition. Ph.D. thesis, Harvard University, 1986.

29. Craig P, Dieppe P, Macintyre S, Mitchie S, Nazareth I, Petticrew M. Developing and evaluating complex interventions: the new Medical Research Council guidance. *BMJ* 2008; **337**: 979–983.

30. Csikszentmihalyi M. Material virtue: Ethics and the Body in Early China. Brill, Leiden, 2004.

31. Cummings TM, White AR. Needling therapies in the management of myofascial trigger point pain: a systematic review. *Arch Phys Med Rehabil* 2001; **82**: 986–992.

32. Daly NP. Hybridizing the human body: the hydrological development of acupuncture in early Imperial China. Masters thesis, Department of East Asian Studies, McGill University, 1999.

33. Fields T. *Touch Therapy*. London: Churchill Livingstone, 2000.

34. Foss L, Rothenberg K. *The Second Medical Revolution*. Boston: Shambhala Publications, 1987.

35. Fukushima K. *Meridian Therapy*. Tokyo: Toyo Hari Medical Association, 1991.

36. Hall DL, Ames RT. *Thinking from the Han*. Albany: State University of New York, 1998.

37. Hammerschlag R, Langevin HE, Lao LX, Lewith G. Physiological dynamics of acupuncture: correlations and mechanisms. In: MacPherson H, Hammerschlag R, Lewith G, Schnyer R eds. *Acupuncture Research: Strategies for Building an Evidence Base*. London: Elsevier, 2007: pp. 181–197.

38. Hammerschlag R, Zwickey H. Evidence based complementary and alternative medicine: back to basics. *J Alt Complem Med* 2006; **12**(4): 349–350.

39. Harper D. *Early Chinese Medical Literature: Mawangdui Medical Manuscripts*. London: Kegan Paul, 1998.

40. Hawking S, Mlodinow L. The (elusive) theory of everything. *Scientific American* October 2010; 51–53.

41. Helms JM. *Acupuncture Energetics*. Berkeley: Medical Acupuncture Publishers, 1995.

42. Ho MW, Knight DP. The acupuncture system and the liquid crystalline collagen fibers of the connective tissues. *Am J Chin Med* 1998; **3–4**: 251–263.

43. Ho MW, Popp FA. Biological organization, coherence, and light emission from living organisms. In: *Stein W, Varela FL* eds. *Thinking About Biology: An Invitation to Current Theoretical Biology*. Santa Fe: Santa Fe: Institute, 1993: pp. 183–213.

44. Hopton A, MacPherson H. Acupuncture for chronic pain: is acupuncture more than an effective placebo? A systematic review of pooled data from meta-analyses. *Pain Pract* 2010; **10**(2): 94–102.

45. Hsu E. Tactility and the body in early Chinese medicine. *Science in Context* 2005; **18**(1): 7–34.

46. Hyland ME Extended network generalised entanglement theory: therapeutic mechanisms and empirical predictions. *J Alt Complem Med* 2003; **9**: 919–936.

47. Hyland ME. Does a form of 'entanglement' between people explain healing? An examination of hypotheses and methodology. *Complem Ther Med* 2004; **12**: 198–208.

48. Itaya K, Manaka Y, Ohkubo C, Asano M. Effects of acupuncture needle application upon cutaneous microcirculation of rabbit ear lobe. *Acupunct Electrother Res* 1987; **12**(1): 45–51.

49. Joepgen G. Integral vision. *Euro J Orient Med* 2003; **4**(3) 4–9.

50. Kalichman L, Vulfsons S. Dry needling in the management of musculoskeletal pain. *J Am Board Fam Med* 2010; **23**: 640–646.

51. Kaneko Y, Furuya E, Sakamoto A. The effects of press-tack needle treatment on muscle soreness after triathlon race — sham controlled study. *JAM* 2009; **1**: 22–30.

52. Kawakita K, Shinbara H, Imai K, Fukuda F, Yano T, Kuriyama K. How do acupuncture and moxibustion act? — focusing on the progress in Japanese acupuncture research — *J Pharmacol Sci* 2006; **100**: 443–459.

53. Kim JY. Beyond paradigm: making transcultural connections in a scientific translation of acupuncture. *Soc Sci Med* 2006; **62**(12): 2960–2972.

54. Kuhn T. *The Structure of Scientific Revolution*. Chicago: University of Chicago Press, 1970.

55. Kuriyama S. *The Expressiveness of the Body and the Divergence of Greek and Chinese Medicine.* New York: Zone Books, 1999.

56. Langevin HM, Wayne PM, Macpherson H, Schnyer R, Milley RM, Napadow V, Lao L, Park J, Harris RE, Cohen M, Sherman KJ, Haramati A, Hammerschlag R. Paradoxes in acupuncture research: strategies for moving forward. *Evid Based Complem Alternat Med* 2011: 2011: 180805. Epub 2010 Oct 1.

57. Leder D, Krucoff MW. The touch that heals: the uses and meanings of touch in the clinical encounter. *J Alt Complem Med* 2008; **14**(3): 321–327.

58. Lee A, Fan LTY. Stimulation of the wrist acupuncture point P6 for preventing postoperative nausea and vomiting. *Cochrane Database Syst Rev.* 2009; (2): CD003281. doi:10.1002/14651858.CD003281.pub3.

59. Lewis ME. *The Construction of Space in Early China.* Albany: SUNY Press, 2006.

60. Linde K, Allais G, Brinkhaus B, Manheimer E, Vickers A, White AR. Acupuncture for tension-type headache. *Cochrane Database Syst Rev* 2009; (1): CD007587. doi:10.1002/14651858.CD007587.

61. Lloyd G, Sivin N. *The Way and the Word.* New Haven: Yale University Press, 2002.

62. Lo SY. Meridians in acupuncture and infrared imaging. *Med Hypotheses* 2002; **58**(1): 72–76.

63. Lo V. The influence of nurturing life culture on the development of Western Han acumoxa therapy. In: Hsu E ed. *Innovation in Chinese Medicine.* Cambridge: Cambridge University Press, 2001: pp. 19–50.

64. Lu GD, Needham J. *Celestial Lancets.* Cambridge: Cambridge University Press, 1980.

65. Lucas, N, Macaskill P, Irwig L, Moran R, Bogduk N. Reliability of physical examination for diagnosis of myofascial trigger points: a systematic review of the literature. *Clin J Pain* 2009; **25**(1): 80–89.

66. MacDonald AJR, Macrae KD, Master BR, Rubin AP Superficial acupuncture in the relief of chronic low back pain. *Ann Roy Coll Surg Eng* 1983; **65**: 44–46.

67. Macpherson H, Kaptchuk TJ. *Acupuncture in Practice.* New York, Churchill Livingstone, 1997.

68. MacPherson H, Thorpe L, Thomas K: Beyond needling — therapeutic processes in acupuncture care: a qualitative study nested within a low-back pain trial. *J Altern Complement Med* 2006; **12**(9): 873–880.

69. Manaka Y, Itaya K. Acupuncture as intervention in the biological information system (meridian treatment and the X-signal system) [First published in Japanese in 1986]. *J Acup Soc NY*; 1994; **1**(3–4): 9–18.
70. Manaka Y, Itaya K, Birch S. *Chasing the Dragon's Tail.* Brookline: Paradigm Publications, 1995.
71. McCraty R, Atkinson M, Tomasino D, Tiller WA. The electricity of touch: Detection and measurement of cardiac energy exchange between people. In: Pribram K ed. *Brain and Values: Is a Biological Science of Values Possible?* Mahwah: Lawrence Erlbaum Associates, Publishers, 1998: pp. 359–379.
72. Medical Research Council. A framework for development and evaluation of RCTs for complex interventions to improve health. Available at: http://www.mrc.ac.uk/pru/pdfmrc_cpr.pdf, posted in 2000.
73. Motoyama H. Electrophysiological and preliminary biochemical studies of skin properties in relation to the acupuncture meridian. *Res Relig Parapsych* 1980; **9**.
74. Motoyama H. A biophysical elucidation of the meridian and ki energy. What is ki energy and how does it flow? *Res Relig Parapsych* 1981; **7**: 1.
75. Needham J. *Science and Civilisation in China — Volume II.* Cambridge Cambridge University Press, 1956.
76. Nishijo K, Mori H, Yoshikawa K, Yazawa K. Decreased heart rate by acupuncture stimulation in humans via facilitation of cardiac vagal activity and suppression of cardiac sympathetic nerve. *Neurosci Lett* 1997; **227**(3): 165–168.
77. O'Brien KA, Birch S, Abbas E, Movsessian P, Hook M, Komesaroff PA. Traditional East Asian Medical pulse diagnosis — a preliminary physiological investigation. J *Altern Comp Med,* in press.
78. Ogawa T. Workshop given at the New England School of Acupuncture, Watertown, MA., April, 1996.
79. Oschman J. *Energy Medicine: The Scientific Basis.* Edinburgh: Churchill Livingstone, 2000.
80. Paterson C, Britten N. Acupuncture for people with chronic illness: combining qualitative and quantitative outcome assessment. *J Altern Complement Med* 2003; **9**: 671–681.
81. Paterson C, Dieppe P. Characteristic and incidental (placebo) effects in complex interventions such as acupuncture. *BMJ* 2005; **330**: 1202–1205.

82. Pickering A. *The Mangle of Practice*, Chicago: University of Chicago Press, 1995.
83. Pomeranz B, Bzerman B. Scientific basis of acupuncture. In: Stux G, Berman B, Pomeranz B eds. *Basics of Acupuncture*, 5th edn. Berlin: Springer-Verlag 2003: pp. 1–86.
84. Puett MJ. *To Become a God: Cosmology, Sacrifice, and Self-Divination in Early China*. Cambridge: Harvard University Asia Center, 2002.
85. Qiu ML. *Chinese Acupuncture and Moxibustion*. Edinburgh: Churchill Livingstone, 1993.
86. Radin D, Stone J, Levine E, Eskandarnejad S, Schlitz M, Kozak L, Mandel D, Hayssen G. Compassionate intention as a therapeutic intervention by partners of cancer patients: effects of distant intention on the patients' autonomic nervous system. *Explore* 2008; **4**: 235–243.
87. Rein G. Bioinformation in the biofield. *J Alt Complem Med* 2004: **10**(1): 59–68.
88. Rochat de la Vallee E. *A Study of Qi in Classical Texts*. London: Monkey Press, 2006.
89. Rugg S, Paterson C, Britten N, Bridges J, Griffiths P. Traditional acupuncture for people with medically unexplained symptoms: a longitudinal qualitative study of patients' experiences. *Br J Gen Pract* 2011; **61**: e306–315.
90. Scheid V. *Chinese Medicine in Contemporary China*. Durham: Duke University Press, 2002.
91. Schnyer R, Birch S, MacPherson H. Acupuncture practice as the foundation for clinical evaluation. In: MacPherson H, Hammerschlag R, Lewith G, Schnyer R eds. *Acupuncture Research: Strategies for Building an Evidence Base*. London: Elsevier, 2007: pp. 153–179.
92. Schoffeniels E. *Anti-chance*. New York: Pergammon Press, 1976.
93. Shang C. The past, present, and future of meridian system research. In: Stux G, Hammerschlag R eds *Clinical Acupuncture: Scientific Basis*. Berlin: Springer Verlag, 2001: pp. 69–82.
94. Shudo D. *Introduction to Meridian Therapy*. Seattle: Eastland Press, 1990.
95. Shudo D. *Finding Effective Acupoints*. Seattle: Eastland Press, 2003.
96. Sivin N. *Traditional Medicine in Contemporary China*. Ann Arbor: Center for Chinese Studies, University of Michigan, 1987.
97. Slingerland E. *Effortless Action*. Oxford: Oxford University Press, 2003.

98. So EW, Ng EH, Wong YY, Lau EY, Yeung WS, Ho PC. A randomized double blind comparison of real and placebo acupuncture in IVF treatment. *Hum Reprod.* 2009; **24**(2): 341–348.

99. Tiller WA. On the evolution of electrodermal diagnostic instruments. *J Adv Med* 1988; **1**(1): 41–72.

100. Tiller WA. On the evolution and future development of electrodermal diagnostic instruments. In: *Energy Fields in Medicine.* Kalamazoo: Michigan, John E. Fetzer Foundation, 1989: pp. 257–328.

101. Tiller WA. *Science and Human Transformation: Subtle Energies, Intentionality and Consciousness*: Walnut Creek: Pavior Publishing, 1997.

102. Treweek S, Zwarenstein M. Making trials matter: pragmatic and explanatory trials and the problem of applicability. *Trials* 2009; **10**: 37 doi:10.1186/ 1745-6215-10-37.

103. Unschuld PU. *Medicine in China: A History of Ideas.* Berkeley: University of California Press, 1985.

104. Unschuld PU. *Medicine in China: Classic of Difficult Issues.* Berkeley: University of California Press, 1986.

105. Unschuld PU. Traditional Chinese medicine; some historical and epistemological reflections. *Soc Sci Med* 1987; **24**(12): 1023–1029.

106. Unschuld PU. Epistemological issues and changing legitimation: traditional Chinese medicine in the twentieth century. In: Leslie C, Young A eds. *Paths to Asian Medical Knowledge.* Berkeley: University of California Press, 1992: pp. 44–61.

107. Unschuld PU. *Huang Di Nei Jing Su Wen — Nature, Knowledge, Imagery in an Ancient Chinese Medical Text.* Berkeley: University of California Press, 2003.

108. Verhoef MJ, Lewith G, Rittenbaugh C, Thomas K, Boon H, Fonnebo V. Whole systems research: moving forward. *Focus Alt Compl Ther*, 2004; **9**(2): 87–90.

109. White AR, Filshie J, Cummings TM. Clinical trials of acupuncture: consensus recommendations for optimal treatment, sham controls and blinding. *Compl Ther Med* 2001; **9**: 237–245.

110. Wiseman N, Ellis A. *Fundamentals of Chinese Medicine.* Brookline, Massachusetts; Paradigm Publications, 1985.

111. Zhu ZX. Research advances in the electrical specificity of channels and acupuncture points. *Am J Acup* 1981; **9**(3): 203–216.

ENDNOTES

1. Much more can be said of this theme. Unschuld describes very clearly the rise of the theory of systematic correspondence in the first acupuncture texts of the Neijing in the early Han dynasty as a parallel to the ordering of society that happened during that time, and as a means to restore order to society (and in the body) following the chaotic period of the 'Warring States' [Unschuld 1985]. There was a clear idea in the theories of acupuncture that they were about providing a means to help restore the natural order of the body that is lost with improper lifestyle, etc.

2. The NIH consensus development conference on acupuncture in 1997 drew similar conclusions about traditional ideas when they concluded that concepts such as *qi* "are difficult to reconcile with contemporary biomedical information but continue to play an important role in the evaluation of patients and the formulation of treatment in acupuncture" [1].

3. Some systems of TEAM practice claim that these patterns are the cause of the patient problems, but this begs the question in the absence of appropriate studies.

4. Discussions and some summaries can be found in Birch and Felt [19: 147–183].

5. Otherwise they would have been clearly observed already.

6. A few papers can be found that have developed systems or information theory approaches to modelling acupuncture [7, 8, 16, 49].

7. Non-penetrating needling can trigger cutaneous polymodal receptors [52], change important cardiovascular parameters [77] and has also demonstrated clinical effectiveness, see the trial by So *et al.* [98]. In their trial testing acupuncture to enhance IVF procedure success rates, So *et al.* inadvertently compared a non-penetrating needle to usual Chinese needling technique [98] by applying both treatments to the same acupoints. The trial is thus a comparison of needling methods rather than a sham control acupuncture study [20, 109]. The non-penetrating needle was more effective than the inserted needling which shows clearly that a non-penetrating needling method can be significantly more effective than a penetrating needle method [17].

8. The trial of Kaneko *et al.* demonstrated that needles inserted to a maximum depth of 0.6 mm is significantly more effective than non-penetrating sham in onset of pain and recovery from pain in athletic performance [51].

9. This kind of needling has demonstrated clear physiological effects [48] and in a trial by MacDonald *et al.* has demonstrated that such shallow needling can be effective for low back pain [66].

10. Including generalised quantum entanglement effects [46, 47].

CHAPTER 3

THE ONTOLOGICAL STATUS OF MERIDIANS

Hong Hai

Senior Fellow, Institute of Advanced Studies and
Adjunct Professor, Nanyang Technological University, Singapore

The "meridian system" (*jingluo* 经络) in traditional Chinese medicine (TCM) theory is a system of passages that transports *qi*, blood, *jing*, *yin* and *yang* throughout the body.[a] It connects the *zang*-organs among themselves and with their counterpart *fu*-organs, and links all other parts of the body including the bone, skin, muscles and tendons and the nine orifices, allowing the body to function as an organic whole.[b] The system also maintains communication between the body and its external environment by carrying information signals as well as energy and materials derived from nature, thereby achieving a balance between the body and its host environment. The meridian system is therefore much more than a neurological network that enables the acupuncturist to treat pain by inserting needles into appropriate points in the network. So broad is the concept of the

---

[a]It is not entirely clear in what ways the blood that flows in the meridians is different from blood that flow in blood vessels. The Chinese is thought to not have differentiated between the two but regarded them as playing complementary roles.

[b]The nine orifices comprise the eyes, nose, ears, mouth, and the sex organ and the anus.

meridian system that the functions sometimes claimed for the system rival in importance those of the organ system.

The meridians in TCM are analogous to roads and highways that link villages, cities, farms, and industrial installations in a country. They have an existence in their own right: they contain *qi* and can become diseased when invaded by pathogens, or they can develop obstructions that hinder the flow of *qi* and communication signals along them. The meridians therefore behave as if they were a parallel system to organs; they can become ill or dysfunctional, and specific meridian-based pathological conditions can be identified.

Because of their association and alleged connection to particular organs, the relevance of the meridians in TCM goes far beyond therapy for pain. For example, acupuncture needles applied to points along the spleen and stomach channels can have a tonifying effect on these organs, hence they are often used for patients with digestive disorders. Acupuncture of points along the *renmai* and *chongmai* are used to treat gynaecological problems as there is thought to be a connection of these extraordinary vessels to the female uterus.

AN INTERPRETATION OF THE MERIDIANS

Among practitioners of acupuncture, a distinction is made between TCM acupuncture and *Western acupuncture*. The latter is used somewhat loosely to refer to acupuncture carried out by those who follow the scientific method established by Galileo and others in the 17th century when they introduced "systematic verification through planned experiments to the existing ancient methods of reasoning and deduction".[1] Putting aside the debatable issue that Europeans before Galileo, and the Chinese before the 1949 revolution, did not use the scientific method, the basic idea of Western acupuncture is that the diagnosis should follow the principles of Western medicine: treatment efficacy should be verified through clinical trials, and physiological accounts should be found for the mechanism by which needling imparts therapeutic effects.

Using evidence-based medical methods, much work has been done on the physiological interpretations of Western acupuncture and on identification of points that can be used for specific therapies. The result has so far been that some of the acupuncture points (acupoints) identified by TCM acupuncture coincide with myofascial "trigger points" but Western acupuncture does not generally subscribe to the configuration, indeed to the existence, of the meridians used in TCM.[2] For pain relief or acupuncture analgesia, biomedical explanations have focused on neurophysiological and neuropharmacological mechanisms. The discovery of transferable analgesia from animals treated with acupuncture to untreated animals by cross-circulation of blood and cerebrospinal fluid led to more intensive research into a cast of neurophysiological players like endorphins, serotonin and encephalins.[3]

In contrast, meridians play a central role in TCM acupuncture as needles are usually inserted into selected acupoints that lie along one or more of the meridians. Historically there has been sustained Western interest in the nature of meridians — whether they exist and, if they do, whether they are neurological networks, paths of low resistance to flows of energy, or the paths for some other kinds of flow. The meridians, conceived as a physical network like nerves and blood vessels, have never been isolated, nor has their biomedical nature been determined despite many attempts by Chinese and Western scientists.

Within TCM theory, there are two distinct questions over meridians that are of interest. The first concerns its role to convey *qi* and blood and its use to relieve pain. Pain in TCM theory has to do with obstructed flow, as captured in the aphorism "Where there is no flow there is pain; when there is no pain, there is flow" (不通則痛，不痛則通). The TCM explanation is that the acupuncture needle stimulates the flow of *qi* and blood. Pain is therefore mitigated by promoting better flow with a needle at the locus of pain or, more commonly, at a receiving point and transmission point along one of the meridians.

The second aspect of meridians is their connection to the organs and their therapeutic use for illnesses associated with the organs. For example, TCM theory would prescribe acupuncture on points along the spleen and stomach meridians to stimulate the production and flow of spleen-*qi* and stomach-*qi*, which are needed to alleviate problems of digestion, bloated stomach, or lack of appetite. This function of the meridians is the more important one for TCM theory as it is an integral part of the overall holistic framework of explanation for illness, diagnosis and therapy.

In the light of the modern TCM concept of the organs as a set of functions rather than somatic structures with fixed loci, the notion of meridians leading to organs becomes suspect, and the conventional maps showing the intricate paths of each meridian with an endpoint in a (Western anatomy) organ could conceivably come to grief (Fig. 1)

An escape from this dilemma is to interpret the meridian maps as being merely schematic once a meridian enters the visceral region, where it somehow interacts with the function of the organ with which it is supposedly linked. This is not entirely satisfactory and a consideration of the ontological status of meridians seems appropriate.

My conjecture is that the intricate network mapped out in ancient Chinese texts, which continues to be used by modern TCM physicians in clinical work, does not exist as a set of physically isolatable pathways. Attempts to map the network using electrochemical and other techniques are likely to be doomed to failure, for the same reason that it does not make sense to isolate TCM entities like *qi*, phlegm and wind for chemical analysis. The meridian system is an explanatory model that experience has

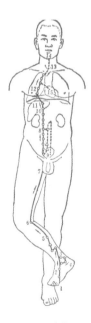

Fig. 1. The path of the kidney meridian as depicted by TCM theory.

found to be useful in the sense that in clinical situations the body behaves *as if* these pathways existed when the physician applies his needle. The biochemical mechanisms, as has been found from recent research on pain treatment with acupuncture, are vastly complex and unlikely to be adequately captured in a system of 12 meridians and eight extraordinary vessels.

As some Western researchers have speculated, the ancients found that pressure on certain points led to pain relief in other areas of the body and, based on their belief in the flow of *qi*, proceeded to map out paths to explain those effects. Over time, these putative paths grew into a large network, parts of which may have been merely hypothesised and not subjected to testing in clinical work. The result was an unwieldy meridian network. One should add that in one of the *Neijing*'s volumes called *Lingshu*,[2] many organ disorders were treated with pressure with fingers or sharp stone implements on acupoints, and a holistic picture emerged which reflected the influence of Chinese cosmological models. These emphasised symmetry and correspondence; in particular, the model of the five elements led to the association of meridians with the *zang*-organs.

The truth of the matter in clinical practice is that clinical acupuncturists constantly improvise new acupuncture points that may not be related to the mapped meridians. These '*a shi*' acupoints, based on experienced acupuncturists' eliciting positive responses from their patients when their needle hits a sweet spot, may have little relation to the meridian system.

To ancient medical thinkers the human body was a black box whose content could only be conjectured on the basis of its external manifestations. Models of the workings of the internal component systems in the black box were invented by observing output responses to inputs. These models were often guided by Chinese cosmology and a rich metaphysical poetic tradition, as well as the belief that the human body was a microcosm of the external universe. Hence an alternative explanation of the meridian is that body has been observed to behave *as if* these discrete pathways exist. We then treat this presumed existence as a convenient tool useful for locating of acupoints for acupuncture. The scientific issue shifts from one of ontology to that of the efficacy of treatments using these pathways as a guide for choosing needling points.

REFERENCES

Filshie J, Cummings M. Western Medical acupuncture. In: Ernst E, White A (eds.) *Acupuncture: A Scientific Appraisal*. Oxford: Butterworth Heinemann, 1999: pp. 31–59.

Kong YC. *Huangdi Neijing: A synopsis with commentaries*. Hong Kong: The Chinese University Press, 2010.

CHAPTER 4

MODERN SCIENTIFIC EXPLANATION OF TRADITIONAL ACUPUNCTURE THEORY

Ching-Liang Hsieh

*Graduate Institute of Acupuncture Science
and Acupuncture Research Center, China Medical University
91 Hsueh-Shih Road, Taichung 40402, Taiwan
clhsieh@mail.cmuh.org.tw*

Abstract

The traditional Chinese system of acupuncture has two main features, namely meridians and points. According to the traditional theory, a meridian is the transport pathway of *qi* and blood. Each meridian system belongs to a specific organ internally, and connects externally to the extremities and joints. Acupuncture at a certain point produces a moderating action to correct imbalances between yin and yang or between *qi* and blood. In the past 15 years, we have designed many protocols and used modern medical devices to verify traditional acupuncture theory. Our findings indicated that (1) acupuncture at the points of spleen and liver meridians induced a change in the mean blood flow or perfusion in the liver and spleen, implying that the meridian system did connect to both a specific internal organ and joint; (2) acupuncture at the left and right Waiguan (TE5) points induced a change in red blood velocity of nail-fold microcirculation, suggesting the ongoing interplay of circulation of *qi* and blood in the meridian; (3) manual acupuncture or 2 Hz electroacupuncture (EA) at both Zusanli (ST36) suggested that acupuncture increased the excitation of the sensory cortex to inhibit sympathetic activity, indicating that acupuncture could modulate and correct imbalances between yin and yang or between qi and blood; (4) 2 Hz and 100 Hz EA at Zusanli induced a decrease in pulse rate, demonstrating the specificity of points; and (5) 2 Hz EA applied to both Zusanli and Shangjuxu (ST37) points increased the natural logarithmic high-frequency (InHF) component of heart rate viability (HRV), whereas 15 Hz EA increased InLF of HRV; these results demonstrated the value of needle manipulation. These findings, overall, provide at least partial modern scientific evidence to support the theory of traditional acupuncture.

INTRODUCTION

Acupuncture and moxibustion include two main features, namely a meridian system and acupuncture points. According to the theory of traditional Chinese medicine (TCM), the meridian system comprises the following: meridian vessels (12 meridians, eight extra meridians, and 12 meridian divergences); collateral vessels (15 collateral vessels); meridian sinews (12 meridian sinews); and a cutaneous region (12 cutaneous regions). Meridians are distributed throughout the body, with each meridian belonging to specific viscera or bowels in the internal dimension, and connecting to extremities and joints in the external dimension. The meridian system is a transport pathway of qi and blood, and the circulation of qi and blood in the meridian system link together as yin and yang, akin to a circle with no end. In TCM, the human body is divided into yin and yang regions, and yin and yang meridians play distinct physiological roles. The relationship between yin and yang includes opposition, waxing and waning, interdependence, and transformation of each other.

The points located in the 12 meridians, and in the governor vessel (GV) and conception vessel (CV) of the eight extra meridians, are called meridian points. In contrast, points located in the extra-meridian region and associated with a specific function are called extra points. In addition, the points respond to the pathological process to form a tenderness point that called the "ouch point," or ashi point. According to the theory of TCM, the development of disease results from an imbalance between yin and yang, or between *qi* and blood, in the human body. The acupuncture needle is inserted into a point to stimulate *qi* and to mobilize *qi* and blood in the meridian. The mobilization of *qi* and blood modulates the balance between yin and yang or *qi* and blood. This effect of acupuncture assists in the healing of diseases.

According to traditional acupuncture theory, a number of factors affect the efficacy of acupuncture, including the selection of points (point specificity and location); the relationship between viscera, bowels, and meridian; needle manipulation; and the combination of points. This paper reports the results of our previous studies, which employed a modern medical approach to investigate these features. We attempted to answer the research questions discussed in the following sections.

1. Does the meridian system link specific viscera and bowels internally and connect to the extremities and joints externally?

We designed a study to examine whether the meridian system links specific viscera and bowels internally, and connects to extremities and joints externally (i.e., "meridian specificity"). Eighteen Sprague-Dawley (SD) rats were studied. The rats were divided into three groups of six rats each. We applied 2 Hz EA to both Yinlinguan (SP9) and Ququan (LR8) points, respectively. The sham group received sham EA at the *Yinlinguan* point, but without electrical stimulation. Mean blood flow/perfusion was recorded simultaneously in the spleen and liver using a laser Doppler perfusion and temperature monitoring system (DTR4, Moor Instruments Inc., Wilington. DE, USA). We found that 2 Hz EA applied to both *Yinlingquan* of rats induced an increase in the mean blood flow/perfusion in the spleen but not in the liver. In contrast, 2 Hz EA applied to both *Ququan* induced an increase in mean blood flow/perfusion in the liver but not in the spleen. These results at least partly demonstrate the specificity of a meridian that links specific viscera with the bowels, extremities, and joints. *Yinlingquan* and *Ququan* are sea points of the spleen and liver meridians, respectively. The *qi* and blood are from sea point of five transports points run into the meridians, akin to the confluence of rivers into the sea.

2. **Does the circulation of qi and blood in the meridian system link together as yin and yang akin to a circle with no end? Is acupuncture at a point locating the target meridian effective? Is the relationship between yin and yang independent and transform each other?**

We used nail-fold microcirculation (NFM) to assess the circulation of *qi* and blood in the meridian. A total of 38 healthy adult women volunteers were studied. They received acupuncture at the following points: right or left *Waiguan* (TE5); right or left *Hegu* (LI4), *Quchi* (LI11) and *Waiguan* of *Jin*'s hand 3-needles; and *Sanyinjiao* (SP6), *Taichong* (LR3), and *Zusanli* (ST36) of right *Jin*'s foot 3-needles.The NFM was recorded in the right middle finger using a Laser Doppler anemometer (capillaroscopy system CAM, KK Technology, England).

The results indicated that the red blood cell velocity of capillaries increased 5 and 10 min after acupuncture stimulation at the left and right *Waiguan*; left and right *Jin*'s hand; and right *Jin*'s foot 3-needles. The capillary density of NFM increased 5 min after acupuncture stimulation at the right *Waiguan* and right *Jin*'s hand 3-needles. After another 15 min (20 min after acupuncture), the capillary density of NFM was noted to decrease again. The results provided support for traditional meridian theory that (1) the circulation of *qi* and blood in the meridian system links together as yin and yang act akin to a circle without end; (2) acupuncture can alter the balance between yin and yang; (3) acupuncture at point that locates the same or vicinity to target meridian can induce greater efficacy because of the right nail-fold is nearby hand large intestine meridian and hand triple energizer meridian; and (4) yin and yang wax and wane, transforming each other.

We designed a protocol to investigate the efficacy of acupuncture in a target meridian or its vicinity. Seventeen healthy adult volunteers were studied. They each received three treatment sessions that included acupuncture at the left or right *Waiguan* point to stimulate *qi*, and sham acupuncture (acupuncture applied to cutaneous portion of left *Waiguan* only). The cutaneous blood flow and cutaneous temperature were recorded on the dorsum central portion of the volunteer's left hand. The results indicated that acupuncture at left *Waiguan* was associated with a greater decrease in cutaneous blood flow compared with acupuncture at the right *Waiguan* point. The left *Waiguan* point and left dorsum central portion locate the same meridian and cutaneous portions of the triple energizer meridian. In addition, both the left *Waiguan* and dorsum central portion of the left hand belongs to the seventh cervical spinal nerve; thus, production of the segmental effect cannot be excluded. Overall, our findings indicated that acupuncture at a point that locates a specific target meridian is effective.

3. How does acupuncture modulate the balance between yin and yang in the human body?

We used the right median nerve short-latency somatosensory evoked potentials (SSEP) and sympathetic skin response (SSR) to investigate how acupuncture modulates the balance between yin and yang. Yin can be seen as representing inhibition and yang as representing excitation; in other words, acupuncture can play an inhibitory role to reduce over-excitation, but may also play an excitatory role to alleviate a depressed state. Thirteen healthy adult volunteers were studied. Electrical stimulation of 4 Hz was applied to the right median nerve in the wrist region, to evoke an N13 component of SSEP at the seventh cervical spinal process, and it simultaneously evoked the N20 and P25 components of SSEP at the primary sensory cortex. The N13 component is a postsynaptic potential of the dorsal horn, whereas N20 and P25 components are generated by two different generators of the primary sensory cortex. Manual acupuncture (MA) stimulation at bilateral *Zusanli* acupoints or 2 Hz EA stimulation at bilateral *Zusanli* and *Shangjuxu* (ST37) points was found to increase the amplitude of the P25 component, whereas no changes were observed for the amplitude of N13 and N20 components, or for the latency of N13, N20, and P25 components. In addition, both MA at bilateral *Zusanli* acupoints and 2 Hz EA at bilateral *Zusanli* and *Shanjuxu* points reduced the amplitude and prolonged the latency of SSR recorded in both palms, as evoked by electrical stimulation of the right median at the wrist. Thus, MA or 2 Hz EA stimulation increased cortical excitability to enhance cortical sympathetic inhibition; the increase of P25 amplitude reflected an increase in cortical excitation, whereas SSR represented sympathetic activity. In summary, we concluded that MA or EA stimulation induced an afferent impulse to the brain, thereby increasing cortical excitation. We furthermore concluded that, depending on the condition of the human body, this cerebral cortical excitation produced an excitatory or inhibitory action by modulating the cerebral cortex. Therefore, MA or EA can modulate the balance between yin and yang, and this modulation is helpful in healing disease.

4. Does acupuncture stimulation induce differential effects between yin and yang in the human body?

According to the theory of TCM, the anatomy of the human body is divided into yin and yang regions. For example, the back and dorsum portions of the hand belong to yang, whereas the abdomen and palm portions of the hand are yin. The relationship between yin and yang is of one opposition and interdependence. Therefore, acupuncture stimulation induces differential effects on yin and yang. For this part of the study we examined 20 healthy adult volunteers. The cutaneous blood flow and cutaneous temperature were recorded simultaneously on the central portion of the right hand dorsum and palm portions, respectively, using a probe (DPT-V2, 3 mm diameter and 1 mm depth) of the laser Doppler perfusion and temperature monitoring system (DTR4, Moor Instruments Inc., Wilmington, DE, USA). Sham acupuncture, MA, 2 Hz EA, and 2 Hz transcutaneous electrical nerve stimulation (TENS) were applied to bilateral *Zusanli* and *Shangjuxu* points individually. The results indicated that 2 Hz EA altered cutaneous temperature in the right hand dorsum portion, but did not change cutaneous temperature in the right hand palm portion. These results suggested that acupuncture induced differential effects for yin and yang in humans. Thus, the essence of yin and yang differs, and they possess individual physiological qualities.

5. Has the specificity of acupoint in physiological function?

We studied the effect of 2 Hz and 100 Hz EA on the pulse of 16 adult medical student volunteers. The pulse rate was recorded by a pulse rate sensor placed on the distal phalanx of the right middle finger. To each/both *Zusnali* point we applied 3 treatments, namely control EA without electrical stimulation, 2 Hz EA, and 100 Hz EA. Pulse rate was recorded for 35 min, including a pre-acupuncture period for 10 min, acupuncture period for 15 min, and post-acupuncture period for 15 min. The results indicated that both 2 Hz EA and 100 Hz EA reduced the pulse rate during the acupuncture period, and this effect was maintained in the post-acupuncture period for 2 Hz EA. The 100 Hz EA did not yield similar results. In the control group (no electrical stimulation), pulse rate did not change throughout the 35 min. The results indicated that 2 Hz or 100 Hz EA induced a peripheral nerve afferent impulse. This impulse possibly evoked neuronal activity in the solitary tract nucleus of the central nervous system, causing a parasympathetic outflow and resulting in reduced pulse rate. In summary, 2 Hz and 100 Hz EA applied to both *Zusanli* points might induce greater vagal activity.

In our previous research, we found that acupuncture applied to the *Shenmen* (HT7) point alone, or applied to *Shenmen* and *Tongli* (HT5) points, induced a lower InLF component of HRV in the post-acupuncture period compared with the pre-acupuncture period. The effect of acupuncture at the *Shenmen* point alone disappeared when acupuncture was applied to *Shenmen* and *Neiguan* (PC6) simultaneously. The InLF component of HRV represents a sympathovagal balance. Therefore, we concluded that acupuncture at *Shenmen* induced a decrease in sympathovagal balance, whereas acupuncture at *Shenmen* and *Neiguan* simultaneously produced an antagonistic effect on sympathovagal balance. Each point thus appeared to have its own specific physiological function, confirming the theory of the specificity of points. Our previous studies also showed that the effect on auditory endogenous potentials (P300) of acupuncture at *Zusanli* and *Shousanli* (LI10) simultaneously was similar to the effect of acupuncture at the *Zusanli* point alone. Overall, our findings provided support for the TCM theory that each point has individual specificity for physiological function.

6. Does needle manipulation affect the efficacy of points?

According to the theory of TCM, needle manipulation is crucial in treating disease by acupuncture. The acupuncturist refers to the constitution of the patient or pattern identification of the disease to select optimal manipulations and points for the treatment. The methods used include twirling supplementation and draining, lifting-thrusting supplementation and draining methods, and directional supplementation and draining methods. Although different needle manipulations are known to generate different results, evaluating the efficacy of acupuncture using the objective quantitative methodology of modern medicine is difficult.

Han (2003) reported that MA or specific frequencies of EA at certain locations of the body enhanced specific neuropeptide release in the central nervous system. For example, 2 Hz EA induced the release of endomorphin, enkephalin, and β-endorphin; 15 Hz EA induced the release of endomorphin, enkephalin, β-endorphin, and dynorphin; whereas 100 Hz EA released dynorphin. These results are highly similar to the efficacy of acupuncture, which depends on the type of acupuncture needle manipulation. Our research showed that 2 Hz EA applied to both *Zusanli* and *Shangjuxu* points induced a greater InHF component of HRV during the post-acupuncture period compared with pre-acupuncture (baseline period). This effect of 2 Hz EA was not replicated by the sham, 15 Hz EA, and 50 Hz EA treatments. In contrast, 15 Hz EA applied to both *Zusanli* and *Shangjuxu* points induced a greater InLF component of HRV during the post-acupuncture period than during the baseline period. This phenomenon of 15 Hz was not replicated by the sham, 2 Hz EA, and 50 Hz EA treatments. The HF component of HRV can be taken to represent vagal activity; thus, 2 Hz EA applied to *Zusanli* and *Sangjuxu* points produced greater parasympathetic activity. This result was congruent with our previous finding that 2 Hz EA reduced the pulse rate. The InLF component of HRV is a parameter of sympathovagal balance or sympathetic modulation. Therefore, 2 Hz and 15 Hz EA applied to the *Zusanli* and *Shangjuxu* point produced different physiological functions. Similarly, different types of needle manipulation cause different effects on physiological action.

7. What is the size or scope of a point?

The idea depth for an acupuncture insert point has been described since the times of Zhenjiujiayijing (published in the year 259). However, to date the size or scope of a point has not been discussed in the literature. Several studies have reported that acupuncture applied either directly to a point or nearby (usually 2–3 cm lateral to the point) produces a similar efficacy. The idea of specific areas, such as motor area, sensory area, and language area, etc. in scalp needle treatment had been widely used in clinical applications. Thus, acupuncture applied elsewhere in the same functional area might produce a similar effect. Our previous research showed that the analgesic effect of 2 Hz EA applied 1 cm lateral to *Zusanli* and *Yanlingquan* (GB34) was similar to that of 2 Hz EA applied to *Zusanli* and *Yanlingquan*. In conclusion, acupuncture applied to a point located in the same segment of a peripheral nerve might induce a similar effect. Further research is needed to investigate this possibility in greater depth.

8.   Does point combination yield a greater efficacy of acupuncture?

The idea of point combination as applied to the clinical treatment of disease began with *Qianjinyifang* (published in the year 752). Our previous research showed that acupuncture at *Shenmen* alone, and acupuncture at *Shemen* and *Tongli* simultaneously, produced similar effects on the InLF component of HRV. However, the effect on InLF of acupuncture at *Shenmen* alone was reversed when acupuncture was applied at *Shenmen* and *Neiguan* simultaneously. For P300, acupuncture applied at *Zusanli* and *Shousanli* simultaneously did not enhance the efficacy of acupuncture at *Zusanli* alone. Overall, our findings suggest that the selection of points plays a critical role in enhancing the efficacy of treatment.

9.   Concluding remarks

We used several protocols to investigate traditional acupuncture theory and to link these theories to modern scientific knowledge, thereby assisting the development of acupuncture science. Our results provided a partial exploration of modern scientific explanations for traditional acupuncture theory. We anticipate that more information of a similar nature will be provided in future research.

REFERENCES

Chou WC, Liu HJ, Lin YW, Cheng CY, Li TC, Tang NY, Hsieh CL. 2 Hz electroacupuncture at Yinlingquan (SP9) and Ququan (LR8) acupoints induces changes in blood flow in the liver and spleen. *Am J Chin Med* 2012; **40**(1): 75–84.

Han JS. Acupuncture: neuropeptide release produced by electrical stimulation of different frequencies. *T Neurosci* 2003; **26**(1): 17–22.

Hsieh CL. Modulation of cerebral cortex in acupuncture stimulation: a study using sympathetic skin response and somatosensory evoked potentials. *Am J Chin Med* 1998; **26**(1): 1–11.

Hsieh CL, Li TC, Lin CY, Tang NY, Chang QY, Lin JG. Cerebral cortex participation in the physiological mechanisms of acupuncture stimulation: a study by auditory endogenous potentials (P300). *Am J Chin Med* 1998; **26**(3–4): 265–274.

Hsieh CL, Lin JG, Li TC, Chang QY. Changes of pulse rate and skin temperature evoked by electroacupuncture stimulation with different frequency on both Zusanli acupoints in humans. *Am J Chin Med* 1999; **27**(1): 11–18.

Hsieh CL, Chang YM, Jin R. The study in effect of Jin's hand and foot three-needle on nailfold microcirculation. *Taiwan J Chin Med* 2004; **3**(1): 14–36.

Hsieh CL, Chang YM, Tang NY, Lin IH, Liu CH, Lin JG, Jin R. Time course of changes in nail fold microcirculation induced by acupuncture stimulation at the Waiguan acupoints. *Am J Chin Med* 2006; **34**(5): 777–785.

Jan YM, Li TC, Hsieh CL. A segmental effect involved in the changes of skin blood flow induced by acupuncture in normal health human. *Am J Chin Med* 2010; **38**(3): 441–448.

Jia BA, Cheng CY, Lin YW, Li TC, Liu HJ, Hsieh CL. The 2 Hz and 15 Hz electroacupuncture induced reverse effect on autonomic function in healthy adult using a heart rate variability analysis. *J Tradit Complem Med* 2011; **1**(1): 51–56.

Lu CC, Jan YM, Li TC, Hsieh CL. Electroacupuncture induces differential effects between Yin and Yang: a study using cutaneous blood flow and temperature recordings of the hand's dorsum and palm. *Am J Chin Med* 2009; **37**(4): 639–645.

Yang YF, Chou CY, Li TC, Jan YM, Tang NY, Hsieh CL. Different effects of acupuncture at Shenmen (HT7)-Tongli (HT5) and Shenmen-Neiguan (PC6) points on heart rate variability in healthy subjects. *J Chin Med* 2009; **20**(3, 4): 97–106.

CHAPTER 5

COGNITIVE NEUROSCIENCE, ACUPUNCTURE, AND PAIN TREATMENT. DOES A STING ALWAYS HURT?

K. Theodoratou

Scientific Association of Medical Acupuncture, Greece
Guangzhou University, China

Abstract

Acupuncture is widely accepted as an effective treatment for acute and chronic pain. During the last decades our understanding of the way the brain processes acupuncture analgesia has developed considerably. State-of-the-art imaging technologies, like fMRI and PET, applied on the brains of people experiencing pain, have indicated that acupuncture controls pain by making specific brain cells more sensitive to the pain-dampening effects of opioid chemicals. Pain is a universal phenomenon with complex biochemical, neural and psychological components. The pain matrix is a multi-faceted brain network that processes painful experiences through its multiple nociceptive and anti-nociceptive pathways. The human brain has the amazing ability not only to receive and perceive our surroundings, but also to manipulate the way in which we perceive them. Cognitive neuroscience and neuropsychology, connecting the mind and body, study the same brain activity, having to do with the transmission, interpretation and — finally — the very perception of pain. Cognition can alter both pain perception and acupuncture treatment effectiveness. The main subject of the present study is the primary understanding of the way our mind and brain manipulate our perception of pain and control the effect of acupuncture treatment.

INTRODUCTION

The human brain is the most complex functional entity known to us. It contains roughly a trillion nerve cells, each of which may make thousands of connections, forming immense networks of circuitry that control the perception of one's own self, and create our understanding and interactions with the world around us.

The functions of the brain and the mind it creates are enormously complex. Everything we do, feel and think emerges from billions of nerve cells and their interconnections. Brain development is shaped by evolution and genetics, but is also greatly affected by experience. The mind is formed through its exposure to people and cultures and becomes a constructive and predictive device. It creates past, present and future inner worlds that allow us to behave in highly adaptive ways, if we so choose. It also allows us to control stimulations, and personalize external messages or treatments.

Several brain regions are activated not only in connection of properties inherent to the stimuli, but also in connection of the psychological reasoning that we perform about them. In a sense, the influence of such reasoning reflects a progressive detachment from responses that are dictated by the stimulus itself and the adoption of information generated by the brain through associations and inferences.

Acupuncture provokes changes in brain chemistry sensation and involuntary body functions: studies have proved that acupuncture may alter brain chemistry through the control of the release of neurotransmitters and neurohormones. Acupuncture has also been documented to affect the parts of the central nervous system related to sensation and involuntary body functions, such as immune reactions and processes whereby a person's blood pressure, blood flow and body temperature are regulated.

WHAT IS PAIN

Pain is a stimulus that follows a certain route within our body, reaches the brain and finally transforms into a feeling.

— Pain is an unpleasant sensory and emotional experience, usually produced by something that injures or threatens to injure, the body.

— Pain begins with a stimulus, but is influenced by physiological and psychological factors before it becomes part of our consciousness.

Pain is something that happens in our mind. The steps of pain transmission are:

(1) transduction at the peripheral receptor site;
(2) conduction along the peripheral nerve;
(3) pain modulation at the level of the spinal cord;
(4) pain perception at the supraspinal site; and
(5) associated sensations, emotional reactions, and effective state.

WHAT IS PERCEPTION

Perception is our sensory experience of the world around us and involves both the recognition of environmental stimuli and the actions performed in response to these stimuli. Through the perceptual process, we gain information about the properties and elements of the environment that are critical to our survival. Perception creates our experience of the world around us, allows us to act within our environment. Perception includes the five senses and also what is known as proprioception, a set of senses involving the ability to detect changes in body positions and movements. It also involves the cognitive processes required to process information, such as recognizing the face of a friend or detecting a familiar scent.

Neuroscience is the scientific study of the nervous system. Cognitive science is the interdisciplinary study of the way information is represented and transformed in the human brain.

PAIN AND ACUPUNCTURE

Science forms the essential basis of our modern medicine. Traditional acupuncture theories, however, are not based on anatomical, physiological or biochemical evidence. During the last 40 years many scientists, both from the Western and Eastern cultures, have proposed multiple physiology models to explain the effects of acupuncture. These models involved endorphins, cytokines, hormones such as cortisol and oxytocin, biomechanical effects, the immune system, electromagnetic effects, autonomic and somatic nervous systems. To date, pain relief is the most thoroughly studied application of acupuncture. Endorphin release at the spinal and supra-spinal levels is thought to be the neurotransmitter effect of acupuncture stimulation.

It is widely accepted that acupuncture stimulates A-gamma and C afferent fibers in the muscles (Pomeranz, 1987). This causes the transmission of signals to the spinal cord, which in turn locally releases dynorphin and enkephalins. A sequence of excitatory and inhibitory mediators in the spinal cord is transmitted to the midbrain through these afferent pathways. Pre- and postsynaptic inhibition and suppression of the pain transmission is the result of the secretion of various neurotransmitters, such as serotonin, dopamine, and norepinephrine onto the spinal cord. On the other hand, the release of adenocorticotropic hormones (ACTH) and endorphins is triggered when these signals reach the hypothalamus and the pituitary gland. Pomeranz's theory research laboratory and other investigators have confirmed his theory with a large series of experiments. Various neurophysiologic and imaging studies over the last three decades provided further proof of his conceptual framework on acupuncture-induced analgesia.

Furthermore, the analgesic effects of acupuncture was blocked by opioid antagonists (e.g. Naloxone). In contrast to the endorphin effects that appear to be short-term, which can last from 10 to 20 minutes up to several days, many acupuncture clinical trials have documented much longer effects. Any muscle afferents or free nerve ending — strongly stimulated — can release endorphin. As a result, the specificity and rationale of acupuncture point locations for different conditions remains unexplained. More recent neuroscientific trials provide that we should study the whole brain network to determine the real effect of any stimulus.

The visualization of anatomical and functional effects of acupuncture stimulation in the human brain became possible only recently, through imaging technology improvements such as: PET scan (positron emission tomography), functional MRI (magnetic resonance imaging) and SPECT (single-proton emission computer tomography). The following conclusions were drawn:

(1) The hypothalamus and the limbic system play a central role in acupuncture analgesia.

(2) The significant overlap between acupuncture and CNS pain pathways suggests that acupuncture stimulation may affect pain signals processed in the CNS.

(3) Traditional needling (with "*de qi*" sensation) and superficial needling activate two different central pathways and yet both provide clinical analgesia.

The main focus of the current neuroimaging studies in acupuncture are merely explorations of acupuncture signal networks, involving the acute effects of acupuncture. Traditional Chinese Medicine advocates that acupuncture can produce long-term effects even though the actual treatment is over. Furthermore, according to a recent study multi-block acupuncture accentuates time-variability and duration. In addition, it has been demonstrated that neural responses induced by acupuncture have excellent time-varying characteristics. Thus, the lasting effects should be taken into consideration in order to study the actual effect of acupuncture. Quite recently, the sustained effect of the acupuncture and its influence on the resting brain drew the attention of several researchers. Dhond *et al.* revealed the intrinsic connectivity of the default mode network and sensorimotor network in the post stimulus resting brain, that can be influenced by acupuncture. There were also reports that acupuncture could exert modulatory effect on the insula anchored brain network during the post stimulus resting period. High temporal coherences in the post stimulus resting state were also suggested, when a set of brain regions are activated by acupuncture stimulation. All these studies and researches underline the existence of various function-related brain networks underlying the prolonged effect of acupuncture.

One common factor of the above mentioned studies is the focus on one or more preselected seed regions of interest (ROIs) and their respective functional connectivity. ROI-based analysis could reveal the brain regions functionally connected to the initially selected brain regions. Still we have been unable to completely identify the joint interactions among multiple brain regions in the entire resting brain networks. Some new research attempted to shed light on the functional correlations formed in the resting brain networks at a whole-brain level. This allows for a qualitative approach to the characterization of the whole entity. It also provides new insight into the topological reconfiguration of the whole brain, in response to external task modulations. The functional correlations within the entire brain, as modulated by acupuncture, were seldom investigated. Acupuncture may induce a reorganization of the functional connectivity across different functional brain subsystems, acting as a peripheral input source capable of transducing signals into the brain. Considering that acupuncture may exert modulatory effects in the entire brain, the holistic investigation of the brain functional correlations should be considered of paramount importance. This will lead to a better understanding of the basic neurophysiological mechanisms supporting acupuncture.

PAIN AND PERCEPTION

The complexity of the brain is not fully described through its structural and chemical composition. The brain is a dynamic organ in a constant state of change, governed by life experiences. Every time we learn something new, form a memory, experience stress or disease, the biochemical structure of our brain is altered at the neuronal level. This affects information flow and is known as neuronal plasticity. Each time, the whole brain network is the real response to any stimulus.

Within a single second, multiple messages arrive in our brain network and our brain undertakes the task to distinguish the most important ones each time. Thus, sometimes we recognize a message, a painful stimulus, but if something more interesting is happening in our brain, then the same message will not be recognized.

Pain is a universal phenomenon with complex biochemical, neural, and mental components.

Pain perception currently constitutes an exciting area of interest in cognitive neuroscience. Specifically, much attention is being directed toward the cognitive ability to alter the perception of pain by manipulating such components of pain as attention or acupuncture treatment, which has been implicated as a significant factor in how painful a particular event or stimulus is perceived to be.

Each single moment brain activity may come to alter, ignore or enlarge the incoming message. Learning, fatigue, movement and other experiences produced by the brain may alter an incoming message.

When researchers applied heat to the skin of all 32 subjects, brain scans using the new imaging technique found that both healthy and chronic pain patients processed the sensation the same way, with no lasting effects. However, when researchers submitted all study participants through pain-inducing handling, those of them experiencing pre-existing back or leg pain, the brains of the patients with chronic low back pain processed painful stimuli differently than the brains of healthy subjects, according to the findings published in the issue of the Anesthesiology journal, dated August 2011. When chronic pain patients raised their straightened legs to an uncomfortable angle for 10 seconds, or performed an uncomfortable pelvic tilt, their pain worsened by an average of 34.3 percent and subsided slowly. In contrast, healthy patients reported no pain during the handling. Among the chronic pain patients, procedures that contained their pain activated brain areas known to process pain, including areas involved in paying attention to important stimuli.

How does a child react to a bee sting? It hurts, cries and feels fear.

How does a patient treated with bee-therapy react to the bee sting? Almost all of them do not feel pain and they expect to be treated and are not afraid.

If you find a spider on your arm, your natural reaction upon discovering it will be quite different when you are certain that the bug is harmless, fear that it is poisonous, or uncertain of its danger. Certainty of the pain intensity of an imminent stimulus is considered a biological trigger of fear responses, which include pupil dilation, accelerated heart rates and, as a result of the opioid-mediated analgesic network function, decreased sensitivity to pain.

Pain does not constitute tissue damage and is not produced at tissue-level. Pain is a function of the brain.

To the extent that we understand the network involved in processing pain, we hope we can use it to provide more targeted treatment that will alter the function of specific areas of the brain. Brain scans might determine who is more likely to respond to particular treatments and also be used to monitor treatment effectiveness.

Not only it is important to describe the constant flux of our brain activity in response to the world around us, but it also constitutes a powerful statement in support of the power of the mind. The mind has (at least from a scientific point of view) an amazing ability not only to perceive our surroundings, but also to manipulate the way in which we perceive them. Studies that explore the placebo effect and certainty of pain relief highlight the ability of the mind to modulate physical activity inside the brain and thus underscore the potential power of the mind. Hopefully, knowledge about the mind's ability to alter pain can be applied to such pressing medical issues as chronic depression and chronic pain. To sum, the realization that our cognitive abilities can alter our perception in ways constituting mere speculation, highlights the intellectual bridge that brings together philosophy and science.

ACUPUNCTURE AND PERCEPTION

Recent neuroimaging studies have revealed that acupuncture stimulation can actuate widespread brain regions, largely overlapping with the neural networks for both pain transmission and perception.

During the processing of a painful experience, other regions process information in circuits that can broadly be assumed to involve: the affective (amygdala, hippocampus), sensory (thalamus, primary (SI) and secondary (SII) somatosensory cortices), cognitive (ACC, anterior insula), and inhibitory (PAG, hypothalamus) regions. Several studies on brain responses to acupuncture stimuli in patients with chronic pain or pain condition, compared to controls, have also determined prominent signal attenuations in the amygdala and SI, as well as signal potentiation within the hypothalamus and motor-related areas. Another recent study has found that the underlying analgesia efficacy of acupuncture mainly involves the underlying molecular pathways, particularly through the activation of A1 receptor.

It is only obvious that a network of neurons, widely distributed across multiple levels of the brain may be involved to the central representation of a peripheral acupuncture signal.

Most neuroimaging studies were primarily focused on the spatial distribution of neural responses to the instant effects of acupuncture. We know that acupuncture needling itself is not sufficient to produce analgesia effects. Both human behavior and studies on animals have indicated that a striking feature of acupuncture analgesia is the fact that it is long lasting: with a delayed onset, gradual peaking and gradual returning. The pain threshold shows a tendency to slowly increase even outlasting the treatment, during a typical 30-min acupuncture session. We can say that the acupuncture procedure typically involves two steps: (1) biochemical reaction to tissue damage through the needling, and (2) prolonged effects following the removal of acupuncture needle stimulation. It is also substantiated that the physical needling stimulus, as well as the delayed effect of acupuncture, can similarly activate many areas of the brain. Thorough interpretations of acupuncture intervention constitute the method of effective characterization of the nature of temporal variations underlying neural activities that give rise to hemodynamic responses, rather than a way to simply detect the occurrence of such changes.

Conventional statistic fMRI analysis of acupuncture has typically adopted the hypothetical approach (general linear model, GLM), and mainly investigated whether activity in a particular region of the brain is systematically related to any known input function. In other words, this approach implicitly integrates specific assumptions or requires a priori knowledge regarding the time to be investigated. Since the temporal profile of acupuncture-associated response is difficult to determine beforehand, this approach is limited and may be susceptible to errors. However, this method still lacks the accuracy to make direct inferences on whether some particular component (brain network) varies over time, as well as the particular time points during which the changes occur. Therefore, great emphasis has been given to the understanding of the temporal characteristics of these spatially-defined brain regions, including considerations regarding the way in which multiple levels of their dynamic activities in concert cause the processing of acupuncture.

Another interesting field is the neural encoding, which is the procedure through which the neuron converts the physical energy of a particular stimulus to electrical activity, finally representing forms of stimulation. The cognitive function refers to all the procedures through which the sensation is being transformed, redacted, combined, stored, recalled or used.

Overall, the results suggested that a long-lasting effect of acupuncture could modulate intrinsic functional correlations in the entire resting brain networks.

Similar results from previous studies have demonstrated the significant modulatory effects acupuncture has on wide limbic/paralimbic nuclei, subcortical structures, and the neocortical system of the brain. The insula presents abundant connections and a functional interface between the limbic system and the neocortex, making it a unique position to evaluate the sensory information it receives based on significance. Should acupuncture mediate the neurophysiological system with more voluntary components of self-control and self-regulation to achieve homoeostasis, then the insula may engage in monitoring the ongoing modulation of acupuncture effects on the internal states of the organism. This connectivity related to the insula suggest acupuncture-sustained effects reflecting its specific modulation on the central nervous system. Another recent study has demonstrated that there is an insula-anchored brain network modulated by acupuncture. Other brain regions, such as the pain-sensory (the thalamus) and the pain-affective (the ACC, amygdala) regions, overlap with the pain neuromatrix.

Therefore, the increased connectivity within these brain regions after the application of acupuncture may describe the specific effect of acupuncture has through the shifting of the autonomous nervous system balance and the alteration of the affective and cognitive dimensions of pain processing.

NEURAL NETWORK LEARNING

Learning within a neural network is called training. Like training in athletics, training in a neural network requires a coach, a person that can describe to the neural network what it should have produced as a response. The repetition is the primary rule of learning. If we repeat the acupuncture treatments, then we will train the brain network to make closer connections and to transform the painful stimuli to a cognitive dimension of a non-painful feeling. Maybe this was the reason why ancient books dictate the performance of numerous treatments, or why in Chinese trials the statistics are always higher!

Knowledge from both clinical practice and from the Chinese books shows us that, for certain pain conditions, we should follow particular point prescriptions and treatment schedule.

Understanding how neural circuits, synapses and neurotransmitters are altered in people feelings is critical in the development of new treatments and prevention strategies.

CONCLUSION

Pain is a universal phenomenon with complex biochemical, neural, and mental components. Pain does not constitute a tissue-damage and is not produced at the tissues. Pain is a function of the brain.

Each single moment brain activity may come to alter, ignore or enlarge the incoming message.

Perception is our sensory experience of the world around us and involves both the recognition of environmental stimuli and the actions performed in response to these stimuli. The cognitive function refers to all the procedures through which the sensation is being transformed, redacted, combined, stored, recalled or used.

Acupuncture provokes changes in brain chemistry sensation and involuntary body functions. Recent neuroimaging studies have revealed that acupuncture stimulation can actuate widespread brain regions, largely overlapping with the neural networks for both pain transmission and perception.

REFERENCES

Bai L, Tian J, Zhong C, Xue T, You Y, Liu Z, Chen P, Gong Q, Ai L, Qin W, Dai J, Liu Y. Acupuncture modulates temporal neural responses in wide brain networks: evidence from fMRI study. *Mol Pain* 2010; **6**: 73.

Dhond RP, Ruzich E, Witzel T, *et al.* Spatio-temporal mapping of the neural correlates of acupuncture with MEG. *J Altem Complement Med,* August 6, 2008.

Feng Y, Bai L, Ren Y, Wang H, Liu Z, Zhang W, Tian J. Investigation of the large-scale functional brain networks modulated by acupuncture. *Magn Reson Imaging* 2011; **29**(7): 958–965.

Huang W, Pach D, Napadow V, Park K, Long X, *et al.* Characterizing acupuncture stimuli using brain imaging with fMRI — A systematic review and meta-analysis of the literature. *PLoS ONE* 2012; **7**(4): e32960.

Kong J, Gollub RL, Rosman IS, Webb JM, Vangel MG, Kirsch I, Kaptchuk TJ. Brain activity associated with expectancy-enhanced placebo analgesia as measured by functional magnetic resonance imaging. *J Neurosci* 2006; **26**(2): 381–388.

Pomeranz B. Acupuncture neurophysiology. In: Adelman G, ed. *Encyclopedia of Neuroscience*. Boston: Birkhauser, 1987: pp. 6–7.

Wang HC, Zuo CT, Guan YH. Research on receptors related to acupuncture analgesia and positron emission tomography radioligands: review. *J Chin Integr Med* 2009; **7**(6): 575–581.

PART II

CLINICAL TRIALS AND PLACEBO EFFECTS

CHAPTER 6

FREQUENT WEAKNESSES IN ACUPUNCTURE TRIALS

Edzard Ernst

Complementary Medicine, Peninsula Medical School
University of Exeter, Veysey Building, Salmon Pool Lane
Exeter, EX2 4SG, UK
Edzard.ernst@pms.ac.uk

Abstract

If we want to find reliably the clinical effectiveness of acupuncture, we need the evidence from clinical trials to establish the evidence. Thousands of such studies are available today.[1-4] Yet we are still far from finding truly conclusive answers. One of the reasons for this inability is that most acupuncture trials are seriously flawed. In this article I will provide a personal view on some of the most frequent weaknesses in acu puncture trials.

RISK OF BIAS AND CONFOUNDING

In on order to firmly establish a link between the presumed cause (acu-puncture) and the clinical outcome (e.g. pain relief), clinical trials should minimise confounding and bias. Acupuncture trials are complex and methodologically challenging. This means they can be particularly vulnerable to various sources of bias.

In a recent review, we attempted to evaluate those acupuncture trials that had been NCCAM-funded.[4] In acupuncture circles, these studies have the reputation for being particularly well-funded and rigorous. It is therefore remarkable that we found many of them to be less than sound.

Thirteen RCTs[5–17] NCCAM-funded RCTs were located; they had been published between 2004 and 2009. In most of these trials, acupuncture was tested as a treatment for a range of pain syndromes.[5–12] Other RCTs tested the effectiveness of acupuncture for irritable bowel syndrome,[13] procedural anxiety,[14] post-traumatic stress disorder,[15] hypertension[16] and postoperative parental anxiety.[17]

Sample sizes ranged from just seven[8] to 570.[7] All RCTs, except two,[8,15] used sham acupuncture in an attempt to control for placebo-effects. Six RCTs suggested acupuncture was effective[5–8,14,17] and six RCTs did not.[9–13,16]

Our review[4] thus suggests that, even for pain management, for which acupuncture is used most frequently employed and where biologically plausible mechanisms have been postulated,[9] the findings from NCCAM-funded RCTs are not uniform: some RCTs report positive results and some negative.

Relatively few RCTs were identified as having low risk of bias, and several RCTs were burdened with major flaws. For instance, Wang et al.[5] failed to publish numerical results: Wayne et al.[6] conducted a pilot study with only 18 participants testing one type of acupuncture against another and concluded that one "may be effective"; a statement which, in the absence of non-acupuncture controls, is unjustified. Goldman et al.[12] applied acupuncture for four weeks, which arguably is too short for generating effects on repetitive strain injury. Hollifield et al.[15] made no attempt to control for placebo-effects, and the authors' conclusion that 'acupuncture may be efficacious' may therefore not be justified. Berman et al.[7] delivered treatments of different duration (26 vs. 12 weeks); the number of treatment sessions in the experimental and control groups were different also (23 vs. 6). This renders the interpretation of this study less than clear.

The influence of the therapist is an important potential confounder in acupuncture studies. It is clearly not easy to blind acupuncturists in clinical trials. This is not to say that therapist-blinding is not impossible. However, so far, very few investigators have attempted to incorporate this feature in their studies and none of the NCCAM-funded RCTs made a serious attempt to control for the influence of the acupuncturist on the clinical outcome. Yet such influence has long been known to be important,[18] and has recently been confirmed in an elegant RCT which, incidentally, was not funded by NCCAM.[19] Similarly, it is known that patient expectation will impact on the study findings.[20] None of the NCCAM-funded RCTs attempted to control for this important variable.

Other frequent flaws in trials of acupuncture include unclear random sequence generation and allocation concealment, lack of patient-blinding, unclear or absence of assessor blinding, incomplete or selective reporting of outcomes, lack of intention to treat analysis and absence of reporting of adverse effects.[4,21,22] It seems obvious that such weaknesses can introduce bias. As these types of flaws tend to produce false positive results, they might collectively distort the published literature and give an over-optimistic impression about the therapeutic value of acupuncture.

RESEARCH QUESTION

It is my impression that many authors of acupuncture trials have not adequately defined their hypothesis or research question. All too often, investigators seem to have just one main aim, namely to prove that acupuncture works. They seem unaware that science is not a good tool for proving a theory but is merely a method for testing hypotheses. Well defined hypotheses are rare. The vague notion "does acupuncture work?" begs a host of further questions which need to be considered.

- For what condition?
- For what patient population precisely?
- What type of acupuncture?
- What dose?
- What treatment schedule?
- Compared to what type of control intervention?
- Efficacy?
- Effectiveness?
- How is the clinical endpoint quantified?

It seems obvious that a rigorous trial requires a well-considered research question. Without it, a clinical study can hardly turn out to be successful.

REPORTING OF ACUPUNCTURE TRIALS

Reporting of clinical trials has received much attention in recent years, and things have improved considerably, particularly since the publication of guidelines such as CONSORT in the mid-1990s. CONSORT-derived guidelines for reporting clinical trials of acupuncture have been published in 2001 and revised in 2010.[23] These developments have resulted in some improvements of the previously dire quality of reporting of acupuncture studies. Yet, a recent analysis of 266 acupuncture trials failed to show that the acupuncture-specific guidelines have been widely adopted.[24] This suggests that the reporting of such studies still needs improving.

Accurate, full and transparent reporting of clinical studies is essential. Without it, we often cannot interpret the results clearly, and interpretable findings are, of course, next to worthless. Crucially adequate reporting is essential for independent replications of trials, and unrepeatable trials offer little in the way of progress.

FUNDING

Clinical trials are expensive and good clinical trials tend to be very expensive. This 'rule of thumb' holds also, perhaps even particularly, for acupuncture. The complexity of acupuncture trials means that they need meticulous planning involving experts in several areas. The nature of the treatment means that, therapists' time needs to be cost. The often small effect size means that long treatment periods and large sample sizes are required to avoid a type II error.

Collectively these and other factors contribute to the often high costs of acupuncture trials. As virtually no potent commercial funders for acupuncture trials exist, the struggle for adequate funding for such studies is frequently unsuccessful. All too often trials have thus to be conducted with inadequate funding, which obviously impacts on the quality of their design, conduct and reporting.

FINAL COMMENT

It would be too easy, I think, to claim that the frequent weaknesses of acupuncture trials are solely due to external factors such as lack of funding or the complexity of designing and conducting a rigorous study in this area. Without doubt, these problems are real and important, but they are not unsurmountable.

A much deeper and more intractable problem for acupuncture research, in my experience, is the acupuncture-researcher him/herself. By and large, this community consists of enthusiastic amateurs who tend to use science to prove that their prior beliefs are correct rather than to rigorously test hypotheses.

When testing hypotheses, scientists conduct experiment after experiment aimed at testing whether their initial idea was wrong. If, at the end, they failed to show that the hypothesis was false, we assume that it was probably correct. Unfortunately this process of falsification of hypotheses has not been adopted by many acupuncture researchers. Generally speaking, the field lacks internal criticism and sceptical thinking. All too often, criticism is seen as a negative attitude and there is too little realisation of the fact that criticism is an essential precondition for making progress.

I suggest that this is a main cause for the many weaknesses in acupuncture trials as well as for the slow progress of acupuncture research during the last decades. I also suggest that, if we wanted to determine the true value of acupuncture, we urgently instil a healthy dose of critical thinking into this field.

REFERENCES

1. Han JS. Acupuncture analgesia: areas of consensus and controversy. *Pain* 2011; **152**(3 Supp): 41–S48.
2. De Gent T, Desomer A, Goossens M, Hanquet G, Leonard C, Mertens R, *et al*. Etat de lieux de l'acupuncture en Belgique. Health Services Research (HSR). Bruxelles: Centre federal d'expertise des soins de santé (KCE). 2011;(KCE Reports 153B D/2011/10.273.05).
3. Derry CJ, Derry S, McQuay HJ, Moore RA. Systematic review of systematic reviews of acupuncture published 1996–2005. *Clin Med* 2006; **6**(4): 381–386.
4. Ernst E, Snyder J, Dunlop RA. National Center for Complementary and Alternative medicine-funded randomised controlled trials of acupuncture: a systematic review. *FACT* 2011; **16**(4).

5. Wang SM, DeZinno P, Lin EC, Lin EC, Yue JJ, Berman MR, *et al.* Auricular acupuncture as a treatment for pregnant women who have low back and posterior pelvic pain: a pilot study. *Am J Obstet Gynecol* 2009; **201**(271): 1–9.

6. Wayne PM, Kerr CE, Schnyer RN, *et al.* Japanese-style acupuncture for endometriosis-related pelvic pain in adolescents and young women: results of a randomized sham-controlled trial. *J Pediatr Adolesc Gynecol* 2008; **21**: 247–257.

7. Berman BM, Lao L, Langenberg P, Lee WL, Gilpin AMK, Hochberg MC. Effectiveness of acupuncture as adjunctive therapy in osteoarthritis of the knee. *Ann Intern Med* 2004; **141**: 901–910.

8. Ahn AC, Bennani T, Freeman R, Hamdy O, Kaptchuk TJ. Two styles of acupuncture for treating painful diabetic neuropathy — a pilot randomised control trial. *Acupunct Med* 2007; **25**(1–2): 11–17.

9. Assefi N, Sherman K, Jacobsen C, Goldberg J, Smith W, Buchwald D. A randomised clinical trial of acupuncture compared wuth sham acupuncture in fibromyalgia. *Ann Int Med* 2005; **143**(1): 10–21.

10. Harris RE, Tian X, Williams DA, Tian TX, Cupps TR, Petzke F *et al.* Treatment of fibromyalgia with formula acupuncture: investigation of needle placement, needle stimulation, and treatment frequency. *J Altern Complement Med* 2005; **11**: 663–671.

11. Deng G, Rusch V, Vickers A, *et al.* Randomized controlled trial of a special acupuncture technique for pain after thoractomy. *J Thoracic Cardio Surg* 2008; **136**(6): 1464–1469.

12. Goldman RH, Stason WB, Park SK, *et al.* Acupuncture for treatment of persistent arm pain due to repetitive use. A randomized controlled clinical trial. *Clin J Pain* 2008; **24**(3): 211–218.

13. Lembo AJ, Conboy L, Kelley JM, *et al.* A treatment trial of acupuncture in IBS patients. *Am J Gastroenterol* 2009; doi:10.1038/ajg.2009.156.

14. Wang SM, Escalera S, Lin EC, Maranets I, Kain ZN. Extra-1 acpupressure for children undergoing anesthesia. *Anesth Analg* 2008; **107**: 811–816.

15. Hollifield M, Sinclair-Lian N, Warner TD, Hammerschlag R. Acupuncture for posttraumatic stress disorder. A randomized controlled pilot trial. *J Nerv Ment Dis* 2007; **195**: 504–513.

16. Macklin EA, Wayne PM, Kalish LA, *et al.* Stop hypertension with the acupuncture research program (SHARP): results of a randomized, controlled clinical trial. *Hypertension* 2006; **48**: 838–845.

17. Wang SM, Gaal D, Maranets I, Caldwell-Andrews A, Kain ZN. Acupressure and preoperative parental anxiety: a pilot study. *Anesth Analg* 2005; **101**: 666–669.

18. Berk SN, Moore ME, Resnick JH. Psychosocial factors as mediators of acupuncture therapy. *J Consulting Clin Psych* 1977; **45**(4): 612–619.

19. Suarez-Almazor ME, Looney C, Liu YF, Cox V, Pietz K, Marcus DM, *et al.* A randomized controlled trial of acupuncture for osteoarthritis of the knee: effects of patient-provider communication. *Arthritis Care Res* 2010; 62: 1229–1236.

20. Wasan AD, Kong J, Pham L-D, Kaptchuk TJ, Edwards R, Gollub RL. The impact of placebo, psychopathology and expectations on the response to acupuncture needling in patients with chronic low back pain. *J Pain* 2010; **11**(6): 555–563.

21. Linde K, Jonas WB, Melchart D, Willich S. The methodological quality of randomised controlled trials of homeopathy, herbal medicine and acupuncture. *Int J Epidemiol* 2001; **30**: 526–531.

22. Ernst E, Lee MS, Choi TY. Acupuncture: Does it alleviate pain and are there serious risks? A review of reviews. *Pain* 2011; **152**: 755–764.

23. MacPherson H, Altmon DG, Hammerschlag R, Youping L, Taixiang W, White A, *et al.* Revised STandards for Reporting Interventions in Clinical Trials of Acupuncture (STRICA): Extending the CONSORT statement. *J Evid Based Med* 2010; **3**(3): 140–155.

24. Prady SL, Richmond SJ, Morton VM, MacPherson H. A systematic evaluation of the impact of STRICTA and CONSORT recommendations on the quality of reporting for acupuncture trials. *PLoS ONE* 2008; **3**(2): e1577.

CHAPTER 7

THE COMPLEXITIES INHERENT IN PLACEBO-CONTROLLED ACUPUNCTURE STUDIES

Lixing Lao,*,† Lizhen Wang*,† and Ruixin Zhang†

*College of Acupuncture-Moxibustion and Tuina
Shanghai University of Traditional Chinese Medicine
1200 Cailun Rd., Shanghai 201203, China
†Center for Integrative Medicine, University of Maryland School of Medicine
520 West Lombard St., Baltimore, MD 21201, USA

Abstract

Recent clinical trial and systematic review results clearly show acupuncture to be more beneficial than conventional standard care in many pain conditions, and basic scientific research has advanced our knowledge of acupuncture's mechanisms of action in a number of pathological conditions. But in spite of the tremendous strides in acupuncture research of the past two decades, evaluation of the modality remains challenging. This is due both to the nature of acupuncture practice and to the inherent differences between acupuncture and Western medicine. In clinical pharmaceutical research, the mechanism of action of a drug is often clear long before the drug reaches the clinical trial stage, and a placebo tablet lacking that mechanism can be designed and employed. Since acupuncture's mechanisms of actions are still largely unknown, it is not easy to identify a sham procedure that does not have actions similar to those of real acupuncture. Moreover, so-called sham acupuncture is poorly defined in terms of location and manipulation. Reported sham procedures include non-needle insertion, shallow insertion at non acupuncture points, the use of acupuncture points that are irrelevant for a given condition, and so forth. Literature review of published randomized clinical acupuncture trials indicates that such sham procedures as needle insertion induce non-specific physiological changes that play a more important role than might be expected from a simple placebo effect that is the result of patient expectations or beliefs. Furthermore, the existing evidence shows that the most challenging issue in acupuncture trial design is the choice of an appropriate control group. While the current research is not without its problems and difficulties, the acupuncture research community has matured, and it is facing its challenges by developing better research methodologies, applying new technologies, and engaging in more creative and innovative translational research.

ACUPUNCTURE HAS GAINED POPULARITY AROUND THE WORLD IN RECENT YEARS

Acupuncture is receiving recognition and becoming popular in the West, and it is rapidly becoming integrated into mainstream medicine in the United States and throughout the world. According to a 2007 survey taken in the United States (Nahin *et al.*, 2009), patient visits to acupuncture clinics tripled in that year (79.2 visits per 1000 people) compared to the numbers shown in a survey taken ten years earlier in 1997 (27.2 visits per 1000 people). Another survey showed that approximately two million adults had used acupuncture in the United States in 2002. By 2007, the number had expanded to three million, a 50% increase in five years.

The increased demand for acupuncture treatment in the West has triggered a vast interest in acupuncture research among scientific researchers and in the Western medical community. In the United States, the research funding provided by the National Institutes of Health (NIH) increased dramatically, from about 20 projects a year in the 1990s to about 150 projects a year in 2007. A similar research effort has been seen in other Western countries, including Germany and United Kingdom, and more recently in some Asian countries such as China and South Korea. A recent review shows that SCI-Expanded indexed 6004 publications between 1991 and 2009 on acupuncture, 3975 of them research articles (Han and Ho, 2011). The United States is the top producing country, China is the second, the United Kingdom is third, Korea is the fourth, and Germany is fifth. On average, 85 research articles were published on acupuncture every year between 1973 and 1997. These increased by 40% in

1998, and the rate of publications has continued to grow rapidly throughout the subsequent years. These data show that scientific research on acupuncture has increased spectacularly around the world, and they suggest that along with the increasing use of the modality has come a demand for sound research on its effects, its efficacy, and its safety.

THE RESULTS OF CLINICAL RESEARCH ARE STILL CONTROVERSIAL

In spite of the tremendous efforts that have been made in acupuncture research in the last two decades, the results of the published clinical trials are still mixed, some positive and others negative; and the interpretation of these results is highly controversial. In 1997, the NIH held a ground-breaking consensus conference on acupuncture in which a panel of experts concluded that there was clear evidence for the efficacy of acupuncture in several conditions, including adult postoperative pain, chemotherapy-induced nausea and vomiting and postoperative dental pain, and also concluded that acupuncture treatment might be useful in such conditions as menstrual cramps, tennis elbow, and fibromyalgia. The panel suggested that more rigorously designed research was warranted to verify these findings. Since then, over 600 clinical trials on acupuncture have been conducted and published worldwide.

Many large well-controlled clinical trials using rigorous research methodology have shown that acupuncture is superior to placebo/ sham controls. For example, a 2004 randomized controlled trial on osteoarthritis of the knee found acupuncture to be statistically effective compared to both sham and education-only controls: acupuncture produced greater improvement in Western Ontario and McMaster Universities' Osteoarthritis Index (WOMAC) function, pain, and patient global assessments compared to sham, and at 26 weeks, the improvement in patients receiving acupuncture was statistically significant in all three categories (Berman *et al.*, 2004). That trial, conducted by Berman *et al.*, had a large randomized sample of more than 500 patients, as well as good controls and an intensive acupuncture regimen. It has provided credible evidence for acupuncture as an adjunctive therapy for knee osteoarthritis, and the results of that study have been corroborated by other researchers. In a 2008 randomized controlled trial in which Jubb *et al.* compared manual and electroacupuncture to a non-penetrating sham control, acupuncture produced significant improvement in pain ($p < 0.001$) while sham did not ($p = 0.12$). The acupuncture treatments provided symptomatic improvements in knee osteoarthritis that were significantly superior to those of the control.

Acupuncture researchers also followed up on the recommendation of the NIH consensus panel that the role of acupuncture in dental pain be more rigorously investigated. In a 2011 study, Lao *et al.* reported that acupuncture performed statistically and significantly better than placebo sham control in lengthening the median survival time between the onset of patients' postoperative dental pain and the time of their requests for pain rescue medication. Interestingly, that study showed a difference between needle insertion sham and needle non-insertion sham: real acupuncture performed significantly better compared to non-insertion sham acupuncture but not to the insertion sham procedure.

Data from another recently published article on pain control, a 2010 German randomized controlled trial on chronic shoulder pain in 424 outpatients, shows that acupuncture reduced pain significantly more effectively than either needle insertion sham or conventional treatment controls at both one- and three-month follow-ups ($p < 0.01$) and that the acupuncture produced greater improvement in shoulder mobility both immediately and three months after the end of treatment (Molsberger *et al.*, 2010).

Several systematic reviews on acupuncture and pain conditions also suggest that acupuncture is superior to controls. In a Cochrane review of twenty-two trials totaling 4419 participants on acupuncture for headache, Linde *et al.* (2009) found six, including two large ones with 401 and 1715 patients, respectively, that compared acupuncture to no treatment and to routine care. Three to four months after treatment, the acupuncture subjects had higher response rates and fewer headaches. In another earlier systematic review, Trinh *et al.* (2004) found strong evidence suggesting that acupuncture is effective for the short term relief of lateral epicondyle pain.

However, in some published clinical trial reports, the data show that acupuncture did not perform better than sham acupuncture controls. In an American randomized clinical trial of 638 adults with chronic mechanical low back pain, Cherkin *et al.* (2009) compared individualized, standardized, and simulated acupuncture treatments to usual care. One week after conclusion of treatment, symptom and function scores for both acupuncture and simulated acupuncture had improved compared to usual care ($p < 0.001$). However, even though the patients in both the acupuncture groups had better effects than did those who received active conventional treatment, the researchers found no significant differences between the real acupuncture and the sham. A German multicenter, blinded, parallel group randomized controlled trial on chronic lower back pain that compared acupuncture, needle insertion sham acupuncture, and conventional therapy followed patient outcomes for six months after treatment and showed similar results. Both the acupuncture group and the sham acupuncture group showed more improvement than did the conventional therapy group. But again, there were no differences between acupuncture and sham control (Haake *et al.*, 2007).

Regarding conditions other than pain, acupuncture may also alleviate such disorders such as insomnia, depression, nausea, and vomiting. In 2010, a randomized controlled trial on acupuncture for depression in 150 women during pregnancy compared acupuncture specifically for depression to acupuncture and massage controls (Manber *et al.*, 2010). Those who received specific acupuncture experienced a greater rate of decrease in symptom severity ($p < 0.05$) and had a significantly greater response rate (63.0%; $p < 0.05$) than that of the controls. Strong evidence for acupuncture in nausea and vomiting comes from five high quality systematic reviews, all of which show positive results or positive trends. In 2009, Lee *et al.* (2009) reviewed forty trials comprising a total of 4858 participants. Compared to sham, acupuncture point stimulation at P6 significantly reduced nausea (RR 0.71, 95% CI 0.61 to 0.83), vomiting (RR 0.70, 95% CI 0.59 to 0.83), and the need for rescue antiemetic (RR 0.69, 95% CI 0.57 to 0.83).

In a recently published Japanese study (Suzuki *et al.*, 2012) on acupuncture in chronic obstructive pulmonary disease (COPD), real acupuncture was found to be significantly more effective than a placebo acupuncture control in improving the symptoms of COPD after 12 weeks of treatment. Patients with COPD who received the real acupuncture also experienced improvement in a six-minute walk test during exercise, which indicates greater tolerance to exercise. Moreover, these patients' dyspnea on exertion (DOE) was reduced. The authors concluded that their study clearly demonstrates that acupuncture can be a useful adjunctive therapy in reducing DOE in patients with COPD.

A 2009 systematic review of forty-six random controlled trials on insomnia, which comprised a total of 3811 patients, found acupuncture to be beneficial in comparison both to sham and to no treatment based on the total scores of the Pittsburgh Sleep Quality Index. Acupuncture was superior to medication in number of patients with a total sleep duration increase of > 3h ($p < 0.0001$). Acupuncture plus medication showed better effects than did medication alone ($p < 0.0001$), and acupuncture plus herbs was significantly more effective than herbs alone ($p = 0.01$). There were no serious adverse effects related to acupuncture treatment in any of these trials (Cao *et al.*, 2009).

WHAT DO THESE CLINICAL TRIALS TELL US?

According to Ernst *et al.*, (2011), which reviewed systematic reviews on pain conditions, out of a total of 57 systematic reviews, fewer than 50%, or 25 of the 57, reached clearly or tentatively positive conclusions that showed acupuncture to be superior to controls. The question is, do those reviews that do not show positive findings suggest that acupuncture does not work or that it is only a placebo? Well, to answer this, we need to look into this question further and more deeply than these studies allow. If acupuncture does not work, how are we to explain away those many clinical trials which show that acupuncture is almost as twice as good as conventional treatment in many pain conditions? And if acupuncture is only a placebo, how can we interpret the results from those many well-designed placebo-controlled trials, e.g., the Molsberger 2010 study, that show acupuncture treatment to be superior to treatment with a placebo control? If the placebo effect and patient expectation underpin the good showing of acupuncture in the treatment of pain, how can we explain the positive results yielded from well-designed studies, such as that of Suzuki *et al.*, (2012), which have employed objective measurements?

Furthermore, placebo theory cannot explain the many mechanistic studies that show physiological effects of acupuncture which cannot be easily dismissed as placebo effects. In human studies, advanced technologies such those that map acupuncture-associated changes in brain function with functional neuroimaging, positron emission tomography, electroencephalography, functional magnetic resonance imaging (fMRI), and magnetoencephalography provide objective means to monitor and distinguish different neurophysiological brain effects. For example, Asghar *et al.*, (2010) investigated the effects of *deqi* and acute pain needling sensations on brain fMRI blood oxygen level-dependent signals and showed that *deqi* causes significant deactivation signals while acute pain produces a mixture of activations and deactivations.

That acupuncture produces mere placebo effects is also contradicted by the mounting evidence of published pre-clinical animal research. The subjects used in these studies, mostly rats or mice, were all naïve animals that had not been previously exposed to acupuncture treatment. Among such studies are those that employed classical physiological approaches of stimulation and lesion of brain nuclei; these show that many brain structures, such as the arcuate nucleus (Arc), the periaqueductal gray (PAG), and the nucleus raphe magnus (NRM), are involved in the modulation of acupuncture analgesia (Zhao, 2008). It has been demonstrated that acupuncture alleviates pain, at least in part, by increasing the levels of all three subsets of opioid peptides, beta-endorphin, met-enkephalin, and dynorphin, in specific central nervous areas, including the spinal cord, the cerebrospinal fluid, and peripherally in plasma. Spinal 5-hydroxytryptamine and norepinephrine are also involved in acupuncture analgesia (Zhang *et al.*, 2012). Further, it has been reported that acupuncture activates opioid peptides and their receptors in the Arc-PAG-NRM-spinal dorsal horn pathway, which act in concert with spinal 5-hydroxytryptamine and norepinephrine to induce analgesia (Li *et al.*, 2007; Zhang *et al.*, 2012). In addition, cholecystokinin-8 (CCK-8) is an antagonist to acupuncture analgesia, which it blocks, and this can account for at least some lack of response to acupuncture treatment (cf. Shi *et al.*, 2011). Acupuncture has also been shown to activate γ-amino-butyric acid (GABA) and decrease *N*-methyl d-aspartate (NMDA) receptor activities to produce analgesia (Zhao, 2008).

WHAT REALLY HAPPENS AS A RESULT OF ACUPUNCTURE TREATMENT?

According to the above described findings of mechanisms of acupuncture, acupuncture seems not merely a placebo (it must be pointed out that like any other medical intervention, acupuncture does have a placebo component in its therapeutic effects). But if acupuncture is better than a placebo how can we interpret the results from those negative studies in which acupuncture does not show better effects than those of a placebo control? To answer this question, we need to understand the nature of acupuncture therapy and the current use of placebo control methodology. In drug studies, both the investigating drug and the inert placebo control tablet are clear in their active, or, in the case of the placebo pill, their non-active ingredients. It is clear that, unlike the drug being tested, the placebo pill does not have an active ingredient that can cause a physiologic response. As opposed to the drugs in these pharmaceutical studies, acupuncture is a physical, invasive modality. Specific active components in both acupuncture and sham acupuncture are poorly understood. Although there is evidence of the physiological effects of acupuncture from the observations of pre-clinical animal research, the physiological effects of any sham acupuncture control (e.g., a needle inserted into a non-classical acupuncture point) are largely unknown. But what seems clear is that the so-called placebo acupuncture is not necessarily inert, as a placebo pill would be.

To better understand the results of acupuncture trials, we need to be aware that a number of different kinds of controls may be used in acupuncture trials and that different types of controls are used to answer different research questions. In choosing an appropriate control group to answer a specific research question, it is important to fit the control to the problem. Three types of controls are commonly used in acupuncture clinical trials: (1) waiting list, (2) non-insertion sham, and (3) needle insertion sham.

WAITING LIST CONTROL

Waiting lists can track the natural history of a disease and assess for spontaneous remissions. Thus the value of using a waiting list rather than a different sort of control group is that the wait provides a way to estimate remissions that may be due to disease variation rather than to treatment effectiveness. For example, in the acupuncture trial on knee osteoarthritis (Berman *et al.*, 1995), a waiting list control group was used. Both patient groups were instructed to continue using whatever medications they were already taking. Acupuncture was administered immediately to one group and delayed in the other group. This type of control was chosen because it offered several advantages. First, it controlled for spontaneous remissions, and it also provided clinically useful information as to whether acupuncture is an effective adjunct to the treatments patients were already using in their actual lives. Moreover, it incorporated an important ethical component in that participants in the control group could also receive the experimental acupuncture treatment. The importance of controlling for disease remissions using a waiting list group was underscored in an acupuncture trial in which 30% in the waiting list group experienced remission of their pain. But obviously the limitation to this kind of control group is that it does not control for placebo effects.

NON-INSERTION SHAM CONTROL

Non-insertion sham acupuncture is also known as placebo acupuncture. Because a placebo is a physiologically inert intervention, placebo acupuncture is only somewhat similar to a placebo pill in drug trials that control for placebo effect. In non-insertion sham acupuncture, a device that looks and feels like a real acupuncture needle but has a blunt tip that retracts into a hollow shaft handle is used to treat control group subjects. The blunt tip touches the skin to create the appearance of insertion, but it is not actually inserted into the body. The disadvantage of this type of control is that it is possible that patients who have had previous experience with acupuncture treatment might be able to tell the difference between the real and a placebo acupuncture procedure. In order to enhance the success of patient blinding in placebo acupuncture, some investigators only include naïve acupuncture patients and exclude those who have previously received actual acupuncture treatment. In studies that employ this type of control, it is extremely important to check for blinding credibility after the intervention. This is usually done by administering a questionnaire asking patients which treatment they believe they have received. Such checking is necessary in order to validate the blinding, that is, to determine whether patient blinding has truly succeeded.

NEEDLE INSERTION SHAM CONTROL

Unlike placebo acupuncture, which involves non-invasive procedures, sham acupuncture involves actual needling, but the needling is done at sites believed to be ineffective for the particular condition being examined. The advantage of using sham acupuncture is that even patients who previously have experienced acupuncture can be easily blinded to treatment group assignment, because the sham resembles real acupuncture. However, since sham needling mimics both the specific effects and the nonspecific physiological effects of needling, the real vs. sham between-group difference may be narrow, especially in pain trials. The non-specific physiological effects of needling can include local alteration in circulation and immune function as well as the triggering of neural pathways such as those that produce diffuse noxious inhibitory control of pain. Therefore, this kind of sham control is for measuring non-specific effects of needling to answer research questions that involve such issues as whether the needle placement does or does not induce specific effects.

Clearly, this type of sham control is problematic. In addition to producing unknown non-specific needling effects, another disadvantage of sham acupuncture is that there is at present no general agreement as to how it should be designed. There is no ancient literature to consult on sham acupuncture points, that is, points that have no specific therapeutic effects on a given condition. In modern clinical trials, reported needle insertion sham acupuncture has been applied by needling at non-acupuncture points adjacent to real points, non-points distal to real points, or real acupuncture points that are not indicated for the specific condition to be treated. Needling techniques in sham acupuncture vary and can involve different depths, e.g., superficial or standard, and various types of stimulation, e.g., manual or electrostimulation. They also encompass a variety of manipulative techniques, e.g., needle reinforcing or reducing; needling angles and directions; and needle retention for various times, e.g., the same or shorter durations than those used in the treatment group. Because of such variations in the way that sham acupuncture is applied, it can be difficult even to compare the results of two sham acupuncture trials that are investigating the same condition. Furthermore, there is no specific research on needle insertion sham regarding its physiological effects in a given condition such as headache or lower back pain: in other words, it is not clear what will happen physiologically to the symptoms of these conditions when a needle is inserted into a so-called sham point. This is in sharp contrast to conditions in a drug clinical trial, since in such trials the placebo pill used is inert and clearly known have no physiological effects of any kind on the given condition being studied. Because of these problems, needle insertion sham control might not be an appropriate control for placebo effects in an acupuncture trial, although this sort of sham can be effective when used for controlling non-specific effects.

DIFFERENT CONTROLS YIELDS DIFFERENT RESULTS

In our review of the randomized controlled trials published between 2006 and 2007 on acupuncture for pain conditions (Meng *et al.*, 2011), in which we compared the various acupuncture controls, we found that the control used might have an effect on trial outcome. Of the sixteen trials using waiting list control for pain conditions during these two years, thirteen of the sixteen came to positive conclusions (13/16). Of the seven trials using non-insertion sham acupuncture controls, six showed positive results (6/7). However, in trials using needling insertion sham acupuncture control, only two of the eight trials resulted in positive or positive trend outcomes (2/8). It is clear that the more invasive controls tend to produce more negative outcomes, and wait list controls produce more positive outcomes (see Tables 1, 2, and 3 in Meng, *ibid.*).

CONCLUSION

Because many factors may profoundly determine therapeutic outcome, the so-called negative outcomes produced by some randomized controlled trials might actually be false negatives due to non-specific responses induced by the control. It is essential to take this factor into consideration when designing acupuncture trials. Careful design and innovative approaches should be considered in order to identify and to minimize such non-specific confounders in acupuncture clinical trials. As acupuncture research becomes more prevalent, it is also important that we researchers become more sophisticated and rigorous. We must remain aware of the complexities inherent in our modality and aware of the factors that make acupuncture research unique. While the current research in acupuncture still has many challenges, our acupuncture research community is facing and meeting these challenges by improving and developing our research methodologies and by applying the many new technologies that are becoming available as we strive to engage in more creative, more innovative, and more translational research.

REFERENCES

Asghar AU, Green G, Lythgoe MF, Lewith G, MacPherson H. Acupuncture needling sensation: The neural correlates of deqi using fMRI. *Brain Res* 2010; **1315**: 111–118.

Berman, B., Lao, L., Greene, M., Anderson, R., Wong, R., Langenberg, P., Hochberg, M. Efficacy of traditional Chinese acupuncture in the treatment of symptomatic knee osteoarthritis: a pilot study. *Osteoarthr Cartilage* 1995; **3**: 139–142.

Berman, B., Lao, L., Langenberg, P., Lee, WL, Gilpin AMK, Hochberg, M. Effectiveness of acupuncture as adjunctive therapy in osteoarthritis of the knee: a randomized, controlled trial. *Ann Intern Med* 2004; **141**: 901–910.

Cao H, Pan X, Li H, Liu J. Acupuncture for treatment of insomnia: a systematic review of randomized controlled trials. *J Altern Complement Med* 2009; **15**(11): 1171–1186.

Cherkin DC, Sherman KJ, Avins AL, Erro JH, Ichikawa L, Barlow WE, Delaney K, Hawkes R, Hamilton L, Pressman A, Khalsa PS, Deyo RA. A randomized trial comparing acupuncture, simulated acupuncture, and usual care for chronic low back pain. *Arch Intern Med.* 2009; **169**(9): 858–866.

Ernst E, Lee MS, Choi TY. Acupuncture: does it alleviate pain and are there serious risks? A review of reviews. *Pain.* 2011; **152**(4): 755–764.

Haake M, Müller HH, Schade-Brittinger C, Basler HD, Schäfer H, Maier C, Endres HG, Trampisch HJ, Molsberger A. German Acupuncture Trials (GERAC) for chronic low back pain: randomized, multicenter, blinded, parallel-group trial with 3 groups. *Arch Intern Med* 2007; **167**(17): 1892–1898.

Han JS, Ho YS. Global trends and performances of acupuncture research. *Neurosci Biobehav Rev.* 2011; **35**(3): 680–687.

Jubb RW, Tukmachi ES, Jones PW, Dempsey E, Waterhouse L, Brailsford S. A blinded randomized trial of acupuncture (manual and electroacupuncture) compared with a non-penetrating sham for the symptoms of osteoarthritis of the knee. *Acupunct Med* 2008; **26**(2): 69–78.

Lao L, Huang Y, Feng C, Berman BM, Tan M. Evaluating Traditional Chinese medicine using modern clinical trial design and statistical methodology: application to a randomized controlled acupuncture trial statistics in medicine. *Stat Med* 2012; **31**(7): 619–627.

Lee A, Fan LT. Stimulation of the wrist acupuncture point P6 for preventing postoperative nausea and vomiting. *Cochrane Database Syst Rev.* 2009; (2): CD003281.

Li, A., Wang, Y., Xin, J., Lao, L., Ren, K., Berman, B.M., Zhang, R.X., Electroacupuncture suppresses hyperalgesia and spinal Fos expression by activating the descending inhibitory system. *Brain Res* 2007; **1186**: 171–179.

Linde K, Allais G, Brinkhaus B, Manheimer E, Vickers A, White AR. Acupuncture for migraine prophylaxis. *Cochrane Database Syst Rev* 2009; (1): CD001218.

Manber R, Schnyer RN, Lyell D, Chambers AS, Caughey AB, Druzin M, Carlyle E, Celio C, Gress JL, Huang MI, Kalista T, Martin-Okada R, Allen JJ. Acupuncture for depression during pregnancy: a randomized controlled trial. *Obstet Gynecol.* 2010; **115**(3): 511–520.

Meng X, Xu S, Lao L. Clinical acupuncture research in the west. *Front Med* 2011; **5**(2): 134–140.

Molsberger AF, Schneider T, Gotthardt H, Drabik A. German Randomized Acupuncture Trial for chronic shoulder pain (GRASP) — a pragmatic, controlled, patient-blinded, multi-centre trial in an outpatient care environment. *Pain.* 2010; **151**(1): 146–154.

Nahin RL, Barnes PM, Stussman BJ, Bloom B. Costs of complementary and alternative medicine (CAM) and frequency of visits to CAM practitioners: United States, 2007. *Natl Health Stat Report* 2009; (18): 1–14.

Shi TF, Yang CX, Yang DX, Gao HR, Zhang GW, Zhang D, Jiao RS, Xu MY, Qiao HQ., L-364,718 potentiates electroacupuncture analgesia through cck-a receptor of pain-related neurons in the nucleus parafascicularis. *Neurochem Res* 2011; **36**: 129–138.

Suzuki M, Muro, S, Ando Y, *et al.* A randomized, placebo-controlled trial of acupuncture in patients with chronic obstructive pulmonary disease (COPD). the COPD-Acupuncture Trial (CAT). *Arch Intern Med* 2012; **172**(11): 878–886.

Trinh KV, Phillips SD, Ho E, Damsma K. Acupuncture for the alleviation of lateral epicondyle pain: a systematic review. *Rheumatology* 2004; **43**(9): 1085–1090.

Zhang Y, Zhang RX, Zhang M, Shen XY, Li A, Xin J, Ren K, Berman BM, Tan M, Lao L. Electroacupuncture inhibition of hyperalgesia in an inflammatory pain rat model: involvement of distinct spinal serotonin and norepinephrine receptor subtypes. *Br J Anaesth.* 2012; **109**: 245–252.

Zhao, Z.-Q., Neural mechanism underlying acupuncture analgesia. *Progr Neurobiol* 2008; **85**: 355–375.

CHAPTER 8

RESEARCH METHODOLOGY IN ACUPUNCTURE

Tat-Leang Lee
Yong Loo Lin School of Medicine, National University of Singapore

Zhen Zheng
Division of Chinese Medicine, School of Health Sciences
RMIT University, Melbourne, Australia

INTRODUCTION

Acupuncture and related techniques have been widely used to treat different types of pain conditions, and this is supported by the fact that 41% of the 3,975 acupuncture research articles published from 1991 to 2009 are related to pain and analgesia.[1] Although there is good evidence of acupuncture induced analgesia and mechanistic model of pain from animal studies, clinical data supporting the analgesic efficacy from placebo-controlled studies is sparse. The impetus for a recent surge in acupuncture research can be attributed to the 1997 National Institutes of Health (NIH) Consensus Development Conference on Acupuncture. The meeting concluded that there is sufficient evidence of the value of acupuncture to expand its use into conventional medicine and to encourage further studies of its physiological and clinical value.[2,3] The formation of the Society for Acupuncture Research also helped to promote and to propose strategies to advance research in Oriental medicine systems, which include acupuncture.

In most Western countries, an evidence base is required to justify the integration of acupuncture into mainstream medicine and the reimbursement of treatments. The concept of evidence-based medicine (EBM) is the application of scientific methods to evaluate clinical therapies not yet subjected to scientific scrutiny. It is the conscientious, explicit and judicious use of current best evidence in making decisions about the care of individual patients.[4] Randomized controlled trial (RCT) is considered the 'gold standard' methodology for evaluating efficacy of an intervention. Most of the clinical studies performed on acupuncture over the last three decades were quantitative research, including efficacy and effectiveness trials. In quantitative research, deductive approaches are used to generate hypotheses and data are then collected to test the hypotheses. Example of questions typical of a deductive approach are "how efficacious is acupuncture in the treatment of chronic low back pain (cLBP) as compared to sham acupuncture or no acupuncture?" (explanatory trial on efficacy) or "how effective is acupuncture in the treatment of cLBP as compared to pharmacotherapy?" (pragmatic trial on effectiveness). The primary outcome measure is usually the severity of pain and / or functional status. Emergent research strategies include qualitative research which employs an inductive method. Typical questions are open-ended without a hypothesis. They invite subjects to contribute to the answers of questions such as "what was your experience when you had acupuncture treatment for cLBP?" Their answers to such questions will then be analyzed, hypotheses could then be generated from qualitative studies.[5]

Common methods used in qualitative research are interviews, focus groups, questionnaires with open ended questions, diaries and reflections. Over the last 20 years, qualitative research has been increasingly used in medical and health research as the concept of medicine shifts from a biomedical model to a bio-social-medical model (especially in the context of chronic pain). This research strategy has brought about a wealth of knowledge pertaining to diseases and suffering and has made a great impact on how medicine is taught and practiced today. We will focus on RCTs which examine the role of acupuncture in contemporary clinical practices, using cLBP as a clinical example. cLBP is a common and disabling disorder and is the leading cause for visits to licensed acupuncturists.[6] It represents a great financial burden in the form of direct costs resulting from loss of work and medical expenses, as well as indirect costs.[7,8] Effective and adequate treatment is an important issue for patients, clinicians and policy makers. Some problems and controversies encountered with current trial strategies will be discussed, and some suggestions for clinical acupuncture research will be offered.

EFFICACY RESEARCH

Efficacy refers to the extent to which a specific intervention is beneficial under ideal conditions.[9] It primarily concentrates on the causal effects of a treatment, e.g. by comparing it to a sham/placebo. An 'efficacy trial' is typically considered an explanatory trial which is performed under experimental (ideal) conditions.[10] While such an approach is typically straightforward in a study of medications, there are a number of issues that make it more challenging to apply to a complex intervention such as acupuncture. As such studies seek to isolate the specific effect of acupuncture in RCTs, the efficacy of acupuncture compared with some form of sham/placebo acupuncture is frequently used. The question of what constitutes a credible acupuncture treatment and sham/placebo control for acupuncture, and what is the magnitude of the non-specific effects of the sham/placebo controls will be discussed below.

EFFICACY RESEARCH ON CHRONIC LOW BACK PAIN

A number of RCTs have evaluated the efficacy of acupuncture (verum/real acupuncture compare to sham/placebo acupuncture) for cLBP. A recent meta-analysis[11] which involved a total of 6359 patients showed that verum acupuncture treatments were no more effective than sham acupuncture treatments. There was, nevertheless, evidence that both verum acupuncture and sham acupuncture were more effective than no treatment and that acupuncture can be considered a useful supplement to other forms of conventional therapy for cLBP. These conclusions were supported by a subsequent meta-analysis from the Cochrane Back Review Group.[12] Furthermore, a recent RCT which was not included in the above mentioned meta-analyses also replicated these findings.[13] The evidence thus far shows that trials comparing verum acupuncture with a sham/placebo acupuncture intervention (whether it is insertive or non-insertive) often report only minor or no differences. The reasons could be as follows: (1) Beneficial effects of acupuncture are due to placebo effects and reporting bias.[14] (2) Sham/placebo acupuncture interventions might be associated with potent non-specific or placebo effects.[15–17] (3) Sham/placebo acupuncture interventions are physiologically active.[18,19] If points 2 and 3 can be shown to be correct, it will be difficult to demonstrate a specific effect between verum and sham/placebo acupuncture.

PLACEBO AND PLACEBO EFFECTS

A placebo, as used in RCTs, is usually an inactive substance or procedure used as a control in an experiment. The placebo can be any clinical intervention including words, gestures, pills, devices and surgery.[20] Most CAM researchers prefer the term 'sham', rather than 'placebo', because sham applies better to research on therapies involving devices, surgery and physical manipulation.[21] The shams that are designed to serve merely as control conditions may actually produce an effect on subjective or biomarker outcomes. These indirect effects of biologically inert substances or inactive procedures will be considered under the umbrella term 'placebo effects'. The placebo effect is a psychobiological phenomenon that can be attributed to different mechanisms, including expectation of clinical improvement and Pavlovian conditioning.[22] Many of these neurobiological mechanisms underlying this complex phenomenon have been studied in the field of pain and analgesia.[23]

Placebo effects do not include methodological factors resulting in improvement that are unrelated to an active alteration of outcome measures, e.g. natural history, regression to the mean,[24] Hawthorne effect[25] — a change in outcome measures solely due to being in a clinical study, such as signing a consent form and having some outcome assessments measured, and poor experimental designs such as subject biases or the purported inert control condition not being inert.[26] The confounding effect of the natural evolution of disease can be solved by including an untreated control group. Proper randomization should take care of the rest. However, unlike in pharmaceutical research — there is no assumption that the control procedure (sham acupuncture) used in acupuncture studies is inert.[18,19] A recent Cochrane review[27] on placebo interventions for all kinds of conditions found that 'physical placebos' (which included sham acupuncture) were associated with larger effects over no-treatment control groups as compared to 'pharmacological placebos'. Linde *et al.*[28] re-analyzed the data of this review to investigate whether effects associated with sham acupuncture differed from those of other 'physical placebos'. They separated the trials in which the physical placebo was sham acupuncture from those which used other physical placebos. Their results suggest that sham acupuncture interventions might be associated with larger effects than pharmacological and other physical placebos. However, there is no evidence to suggest that sham acupuncture interventions involving skin penetration are associated with larger non-specific effects than those which do not.[17,29] The evidence thus far suggests that sham acupuncture control (invasive/non-invasive) is associated with an enhanced placebo effect compared to other physical and pharmacological placebos. In addition, Linde *et al.*[17] performed another systematic review of acupuncture trials in any condition including both sham and no-treatment groups. Their primary aim was to investigate the size of non-specific effects of acupuncture (difference between sham acupuncture vs. no acupuncture). Their secondary aims were to investigate factors (such as type of sham intervention, condition, study quality or intensity of co-interventions) possibly influencing the size of such non-specific effects and to quantify the specific (difference between acupuncture vs. sham acupuncture) and total effects of acupuncture (difference between acupuncture vs. no acupuncture) in the included trials. They concluded that sham acupuncture interventions are often associated with moderately large non-specific effects, which could make it difficult to detect a small additional specific effect when comparing verum acupuncture and sham acupuncture.

The evidence so far shows that sham acupuncture is associated with an enhanced non-specific effect (including placebo effect), and this enhanced effect can be further reinforced by patients' expectations.[30,31] It has been shown that patients with higher expectations about acupuncture treatment experienced larger clinical improvements than patients with lower expectations, regardless of the allocation to real acupuncture or sham acupuncture. Thus it did not really matter whether the patients actually received the real or the sham procedure. What mattered was whether they believed in acupuncture and expected a benefit from it. Interestingly, a significant difference between patients with low and those with high expectations was still detected when followed-up at six months, which indicates powerful long-lasting effects.[30]

Benedetti[32] suggests that research on placebo mechanisms has at least two important implications for clinical trials: (1) The design of protocols that circumvent the need of a placebo arm. An example is the "open/hidden" protocol, where the placebo component stands out as the difference between overt or covert drug administration, with no patients receiving sham treatment. This approach is obviously not applicable to acupuncture research (2) The re-evaluation of clinical trial methodology. Patient expectations are not usually among the controlled variables but they have the potential to differentially influence improvement in both control (placebo) and drug arms, thus invalidating the attempt at separating the pharmacodynamic effect. Studies on acupuncture have showed that results could be drastically reversed by redistributing the participants according to what they believed was their group of assignment.[30,31] In other words, no differences were found with the standard grouping, but the participants expecting real acupuncture reported significant less pain than those believing to be in the sham group, regardless of the real assignment.

SHAM ACUPUNCTURE INTERVENTIONS ARE PHYSIOLOGICALLY ACTIVE

A variety of different placebo controls have been used in acupuncture clinical trials. Birch[33] has reviewed the literatures and explored ten research models for conducting sham-controlled trials of acupuncture. He also discussed the merit and demerit of each model in terms of matching the non-specific effects associated with acupuncture treatment. Four main types of sham acupuncture were commonly used based on needling (with/ without skin penetration) and point selection (therapeutic point indicated for the condition, acupuncture point not indicated for the condition, and 'non-acupuncture point'/'sham point'):

(1) Skin penetrating — (a) insertion or superficial insertion at true acupuncture points without further stimulation (e.g. to obtain *deqi* feeling), it was felt that this form of sham control will carry therapeutic effect and should be avoided, (b) insertion or superficial insertion at non-acupuncture points with minimal stimulation. This is the most popular form of control used. However, needles inserted into non-acupuncture points and/or superficially used as sham control may not necessarily inert and may have both specific and non-specific effects.[18] In addition, it remains uncertain what constitutes a valid non-acupuncture point/sham point, e.g. true points unrelated to the condition being treated or points located a short distance away from the true points (but located on an area with no known meridian).

(2) Non-skin penetrating — (a) non-insertion at non-acupuncture points, (b) non-insertion at true acupuncture points. Non-skin penetrating devices include the use of blunt end of a cocktail stick, needle's guide tube, tooth prick, and retractable needle (needle has a blunt tip and retracts into a hollow shaft handle).[34,35]

Non-insertion devices were introduced to avoid skin penetration, hence any physiological effects associated with needling should be minimized. However, evidence so far suggests that both invasive and non-invasive devices can produce the same degree of non-specific effect during acupuncture trials (i.e. non-insertion devices are not physiologically inert).[17,29] Historically and clinically, acupuncture intervention can be carried out with non-invasive techniques[36] and non-insertion devices have been available for many centuries. A recent Cochrane review[37] concluded that touch therapies (including healing touch and Reiki) may have a modest effect in pain relief. Kerr and colleagues noted that there are many important common factors shared by touch healing and sham acupuncture rituals (e.g. touch stimulation, the meaning attached to the touch and the modulation of the patient's own somatosensory attention to touch). They conducted a qualitative study[38] by interviewing a subset of acupuncture naïve patients involved in a single-blind RCT in IBS,[39] to describe their treatment experiences while undergoing a course of sham acupuncture treatment. Their results showed that in five of six cases, patients associated sensations including 'warmth' and 'tingling' with treatment efficacy. Similar touch sensations were also reported by patients in previous accounts of ritual touch healing. In addition, their patients described their experiences with such touch sensations as motivating their belief in the practitioner's ability to tailor treatments to patients' specific conditions.

STRENGTH AND WEAKNESSES OF ACUPUNCTURE EFFICACY RESEARCH

The main strength of RCT is to preclude biases such as selection bias (by randomizing patients to groups and by concealing the allocation), observation bias (by blinding doctors and patients), and reporting bias (by blinding outcome assessors and statisticians). Although RCTs provide essential, high-quality evidence about the benefits and harms of medical interventions, many such trials have limited relevance to clinical practice. The investigations are often structured in ways that fail to address patients' and clinicians' actual questions about a given treatment. Efficacy trials dictate that the investigators enroll a homogeneous patient population (with strict inclusion and exclusion criteria), prescribe a standard treatment for all the trial subjects to be followed strictly, and inform neither patients nor study personnel about treatment assignments. Thus, although these trials are conducted in clinical settings, their enrolled populations and treatment approaches do not reflect the complexity and diversity of actual clinical practice such as acupuncture.

Pharmacologic intervention trials generally involve a specific inhibitor, enhancer, or modifier for a specific, known pathway to be modified. In contrast, although the neurophysiological mechanisms of acupuncture induced analgesia are quite well established in research for experimental pain, the exact mechanisms underlying the action of acupuncture in clinical practice for chronic pain conditions is still unclear. Walach[40] warned against the use of the existing RCT model to study complementary and alternative medicine such as acupuncture, as both the verum and sham acupuncture have been shown to generate a large non-specific effects, hence, any potential specific effects were overlooked in most studies which were likely to be under-powered. The explanations as to why many efficacy trials could not demonstrate a difference between verum and sham acupuncture are: (1) The actual mechanism(s) of acupuncture induced analgesia is still unknown, it is likely to involve multiple mechanisms acting locally (painful site), as well as at the spinal and supra-spinal levels. Hence, a credible placebo control for acupuncture is not possible until we can elicit the mechanisms of action of acupuncture. (2) Sham controls are physiologically active,[18,19,38] and are also associated with potent non-specific or placebo effects.[15–17,39] If sham control is not inert, sham-controlled trials of acupuncture can be viewed as comparing one form of treatment against another. Further, sham acupuncture points commonly chosen are often located in the same neural segments as the real acupuncture points (i.e. same dermatomes or myotomes). These sham points could be considered as real acupuncture points, or therapeutic points. (3) There is strong evidence to show that the endogenous opioid system is activated by acupuncture[41] as well as placebo control.[23] Hence, the possibility of a type 2 (false-negative) error in many acupuncture efficacy trials cannot be ruled out.[40,42]

EFFECTIVENESS RESEARCH

"Effectiveness" is a "measure of the extent to which an intervention, when deployed in the field in routine circumstances, does what it is intended to do for a specific population".[9] In other words "effectiveness" reflects whether a treatment is beneficial under conditions close to routine care and such effectiveness studies are also known as "pragmatic" or "practical" trials. RCTs can be efficacy (explanatory) or effectiveness (pragmatic) trials. Pragmatic trials (PTs) are designed and conducted to answer important questions facing patients, clinicians, and policy makers. The characteristic features of PTs are that they (1) select clinically relevant alternative interventions to compare, (2) include a diverse population of study participants, (3) recruit participants from heterogeneous practice settings, and (4) collect data on a broad range of health outcomes.[43] PTs compare two or more medical interventions that are directly relevant to clinical care or health care delivery (e.g. acupuncture vs. physiotherapy), and strive to assess those interventions' effectiveness in real-world practice. However, since neither providers nor patients were blinded to treatment, an observation bias cannot be ruled out.

EFFECTIVENESS RESEARCH ON CHRONIC LOW BACK PAIN

PTs have been reported in which the effectiveness of acupuncture was evaluated against standard care, or as an overall effect of an additional acupuncture treatment against standard care alone. In addition, these studies also looked into the issue of cost-effectiveness of acupuncture, based on the quality-adjusted life year's measurement. A pragmatic, two-parallel group, RCT involving 230 patients was reported in UK.[44] Patients in the experimental arm were offered the option of referral to the acupuncture service. The control group received usual care from their general practitioner (commonly entailed a mixture of physiotherapy, medication and recommended back exercises). The trial protocol allowed up to ten individualized acupuncture treatments per patient. The acupuncturists determined the content and the number of treatments according to patients' need. The result showed that acupuncture care and usual care were both associated with clinically significant improvement at 12- and 24-month follow-up. However, acupuncture care was significantly more effective in reducing bodily pain than usual care at 24-month follow-up. In addition, the acupuncture service was found to be cost-effective at 24 months. Although the National Health Service costs were greater in the acupuncture care group than in the usual care group, the additional resource use was less than the costs of the acupuncture treatment itself, suggesting that some usual care resource use was offset.

Another study involving more than eleven thousands patients was carried out in Germany.[45] Patients with cLBP were allocated to an acupuncture group or a no- acupuncture control group. Patients who did not consent to randomization were included in a non-randomized acupuncture group. All patients were allowed to receive routine medical care in addition to study treatment. The result showed that acupuncture carried out on randomized patients as well as on non-randomized patients, in addition to routine care, resulted in a clinically relevant benefit and was cost-effective among patients with cLBP from primary care practices in Germany.

RESEARCH ON INTERVENTIONAL THERAPIES FOR PAIN MANAGEMENT IN ORTHODOX MEDICINE

Theoretically, none of the pain management studies are supported by a high level of evidence. We will cite two examples to illustrate the dilemma and controversy concerning efficacy and effectiveness research involving the use of invasive techniques in orthodox medicine and its relevance to acupuncture research.

(1) Epidural steroid injections have been used for more than 50 years to treat low back pain and are the most common intervention in pain clinics throughout the world.[46] Yet despite their widespread use, their efficacy is unclear. A recent updated Cochrane review concluded that there is insufficient evidence to support the use of injection therapy in subacute and chronic low back pain.[47] However, Benyamin *et al.*[48] and Manchikanti *et al.*[49] carried out systematic reviews on RCTs (with no sham control) evaluating the effectiveness of lumbar interlaminar and lumbar transforaminal epidural steroid injections respectively in managing lumbar spinal pain. They concluded that there is fair to good evidence to support the use of epidural steroid injections by the above mentioned routes in managing spinal pain of different etiologies. These authors also emphasize that placebo-controlled neural blockade is not realistic, and that the underlying mechanism of action of epidurally administered steroid and local anesthetic injection is still not well understood. Cohen[50] is also of the opinion that after thirty-five studies or so have failed to provide a definitive answer regarding the efficacy of epidural steroid injections, it is unlikely that future trials will do so.

(2) Vertebroplasty (vertebral augmentation), an invasive procedure which involves injecting liquid cement through a needle into the vertebral body, where it hardens and is thought to restore stability, has been widely used to treat painful, osteoporotic vertebral compression fractures.[51] Two recent RCTs conducted by two independent groups, using sham surgery as control (efficacy trials), have found no beneficial effect (vertebroplasty is a placebo effect).[52,53] However, RCTs comparing vertebral augmentation with conventional medical therapy (pragmatic trials) showed augmentation to be beneficial.[54–56]

Taken together, it seems that efficacy trials involving many physical interventions may share the similar dilemma of acupuncture. However, there are fundamental differences between acupuncture and physical interventions that are derived from knowledge of Western medical science (e.g. epidural steroid injections and vertebroplasty). Furthermore, traditional acupuncture, as part of Chinese medicine, is understood to be a form of holistic medicine, which addresses not only the pain symptom, but also takes care of the root cause based on Chinese medicine diagnosis. Chinese medicine, together with other complementary and alternative medicines such as Ayurveda or homeopathy, is classified as whole medical systems. The National Center for Complementary and Alternative Medicine defines whole medical systems as systems that are built upon complete systems of theory and practice. Such systems have evolved prior and separate from the conventional medical approach.[57] Clinical research on whole medical systems is confronted with two major disadvantages: (1) a fragmentation of their treatment, and (2) interventions which follow a Western diagnostic approach. Pragmatic studies focusing on effectiveness and including additional aspects of the traditional diagnosis could help overcome these problems.[58]

CONCLUSION AND SUMMARY OF THE CURRENT STATUS OF ACUPUNCTURE AND CLBP

In view of the complex pathophysiology of many chronic pain conditions including cLBP, the lack of a credible sham control, and a strong placebo effect associated with the use of invasive technique, we consider the differences between efficacy and effectiveness studies reflect the differences in assessing the components of acupuncture or the whole effect of acupuncture. Instead, we should concentrate on doing more pragmatic studies focusing on the effectiveness and to include additional aspects of the traditional diagnosis on various types of chronic pain conditions. This sentiment is also shared by pain management physicians using interventional techniques to treat chronic pain conditions.[48,49] When the relevant clinical trials are not available (e.g. cLBP), pragmatic trials have the potential to be an important source of information to guide clinical practice and health care delivery.[59-61]

Li and Kaptchuk62 expressed in a recent editorial that in our current cost-conscious environment, especially when other effective and safe clinical options are unavailable, policy makers put effectiveness above efficacy. This shift may represent a societal shift in which regulatory and insurance bodies and "patient-centered health care" have begun to outweigh the "evidence-based medicine" of researchers in determining an intervention's legitimacy. Further, Ambrósio *et al.*[63] found that acupuncture appears to be a cost-effective intervention for some chronic pain conditions including cLBP. They reviewed seven cost-utility studies and showed that the cost per quality adjusted life year gained to be below typical thresholds of willingness to pay. Currently, acupuncture is being recommended for the treatment of cLBP by some policy makers and professional organizations — the German Federal Committee of Physicians and Health Insurers,[64] the National Institute for Health and Clinical Excellence (NICE),[64] and the American College of Physicians and the American Pain Society.[66]

REFERENCES

1. Han JS, Ho YS. Global trends and performances of acupuncture research. *Neurosci Biobehav Rev* 2011; **35**: 680–687.
2. NIH Consensus Conference. Acupuncture. *JAMA* 1998; **280**: 1518–1524.
3. Langevin HM, Wayne PM, Macpherson H, *et al.* Paradoxes in acupuncture research: strategies for moving forward. *Evid Based Compl Alt Med* 2011; **2011**: 1–11.
4. Sackett DL, Rosenberg WM, Gray JA, Haynes RB, Richardson WS. Evidence-based medicine: what it is and what it isn't. *BMJ* 1996; **312**: 71–72.
5. Bourgeault IL, Dingwall R, De Vries R. Introduciton. In: Bourgeault IL, Dingwall R, De Vries R, eds. *The Sage Handbook of Qualitative Methods in Health Research*. London: Sage Publications Ltd. 2010: pp. 1–16.
6. Cherkin DC, Deyo RA, Sherman KJ, *et al.* Characteristics of visits to licensed acupuncturists, chiropractors, massage therapists, and naturopathic physicians. *J Am Board Fam Pract* 2002; **15**: 463–472.
7. Frymoyer JW, Cats-Baril WL. An overview of the incidences and costs of low back pain. *Orthop Clin North Am* 1991; **22**: 263–271.

8. Von Korff M, Ormel J, Keefe FJ, Dworkin SF. Grading the severity of chronic pain. *Pain* 1992; **50**: 133–149.

9. Last J, Spasoff, RA, Harris S. *A Dictionary of Epidemiology*. 4th ed. Oxford: Oxford University Press, 2001.

10. Witt CM. Efficacy, effectiveness, pragmatic trials — guidance on terminology and the advantages of pragmatic trials. *Forsch Komplementärmed Klass Naturheilkd* 2009; **16**: 292–294.

11. Yuan J, Purepong N, Kerr DP, Park J, Bradbury I, McDonough S. Effectiveness of acupuncture for low back pain: a systematic review. *Spine* 2008; **33**: E887–E900.

12. Rubinstein SM, van Middelkoop M, Kuijpers T, *et al.* A systematic review on the effectiveness of complementary and alternative medicine for chronic non-specific low-back pain. *Eur Spine J* 2010; **19**: 1213–1228.

13. Cherkin D, Sherman KJ, Avins AL, *et al.* A randomized trial comparing acupuncture, simulated acupuncture, and usual care for chronic low back pain. *Arch Intern Med* 2009; **169**: 858–866.

14. Bausell RB: *Snake oil science: The Truth about Complementary and Alternative Medicine*. Oxford, UK: Oxford University Press; 2007.

15. Kaptchuk TJ. The placebo effect in alternative medicine: can the performance of a healing ritual have clinical significance? *Ann Intern Med* 2002, **136**: 817–825.

16. Liu T, Yu CP. Placebo analgesia, acupuncture and sham surgery. *Evid Based Compl Alt Med* 2011; **2011**: 943–947

17. Linde K, Niemann K, Schneider A, Meissner K. How large are the non-specific effects of acupuncture? A meta-analysis of randomized controlled trials. *BMC Med* 2010; **8**: 75.

18. Birch S. A review and analysis of placebo treatments, placebo effects, and placebo controls in trials of medical procedures when sham is not inert. *J Alternat Complement Med* 2006; **12**: 303–310.

19. Lund I, Lundeberg T. Are minimal, superficial or sham acupuncture procedures acceptable as inert placebo controls? *Acupunct Med* 2006, **24**: 13–15.

20. Chaput de Saintonge DM, Herxheimer A. Harnessing placebo effects in health care. *Lancet* 1994; **344**: 995–998.

21. Hammerschlag R, Zwickey H. Evidence-based complementary and alternative medicine: back to basics. *J Alternat Complement Med* 2006; **12**: 349–350.

22. Oken BS. Placebo effects: clinical aspects and neurobiology. *Brain* 2008; **131**: 2812–2823.

23. Benedetti F, Mayberg HS, Wager TD, Stohler CS, Zubieta JK. Neurobiological mechanisms of the placebo effect. *J Neurosci* 2005; **25**: 10390–10402.

24. McDonald CJ, Mazzuca SA. How much of the placebo 'effect' is really statistical regression? *Stat Med* 1983; **2**: 417–427.

25. Bouchet C, Guillemin F, Briancon S. Non-specific effects in longitudinal studies: impact on quality of life measures. *J Clin Epidemiol* 1996; **49**: 15–20.

26. Kienle GS, Kiene H. The powerful placebo effect: fact or fiction? *J Clin Epidemiol* 1997; **50**: 1311–1318.

27. Hrobjartsson A, Gotzsche PC. Placebo interventions for all clinical conditions. *Cochrane Database Syst Rev* 2010; CD003974.

28. Linde K, Niemann K, Meissner K. Are sham acupuncture interventions more effective than (other) placebos? A re-analysis of data from the Cochrane review on placebo effects. *Forsch Komplementmed* 2010; **17**: 259–264.

29. Madsen MV, Gøtzsche PC, Hrobjartsson A. Acupuncture treatment for pain: systematic review of randomised clinical trials with acupuncture, placebo acupuncture, and no acupuncture groups. *BMJ* 2009; **338**: 330–333.

30. Linde K, Witt CM, Streng A *et al.* The impact of patient expectations on outcomes in four randomized controlled trials of acupuncture in patients with chronic pain. *Pain* 2007; **128**: 264–271.

31. Bausell RB, Lao L, Bergman S, Lee WL, Berman BM. Is acupuncture analgesia an expectancy effect? Preliminary evidence based on participants' perceived assignments in two placebo-controlled trials. *Eval Health Prof* 2005; **28**: 9–26.

32. Benedetti F. Placebo-induced improvements: how therapeutic rituals affect the patient's brain. *J Acupunct Meridian Stud* 2012; **5**: 97–103.

33. Birch S. Controlling for non-specific effects of acupuncture in clinical trials. *Clini Acupunct Oriental Med* 2003; **4**: 59–70.

34. Streitberger K, Kleinhenz J. Introducing a placebo needle into acupuncture research. *Lancet* 1998; **352**: 364–365.

35. Park J, White A, Stevinson C, Ernst E, James M. Validating a new non-penetrating sham acupuncture device: two randomised controlled trials. *Acupunct Med* 2002; **20**: 168–174.

36. *WHO. Guidelines for Clinical Research on Acupuncture*. Western Pacific: WHO Regional Publications, 1995: pp. 66.

37. So PS, Jiang Y, Qin Y. Touch therapies for pain relief in adults. *Cochrane Database Syst Rev* 2008; **4**: CD006535.

38. Kerr CE, Shaw JR, Conboy LA, Kelley JM, Jacobson E, Kaptchuk TJ. Placebo acupuncture as a form of ritual touch healing: a neurophenomenological model. *Conscious Cogn* 2011; **20**: 784–791.

39. Kaptchuk TJ, Kelley JM, Conboy LA, *et al.* Components of placebo effect: randomised controlled trial in patients with irritable bowel syndrome. *BMJ* 2008; **336**: 999–1003.

40. Walach H. The efficacy paradox in randomized controlled trials of CAM and elsewhere: beware of the placebo trap. *J Altern Complement Med* 2001; **7**: 213–218.

41. Han JS. Acupuncture and endorphins. *Neurosci Lett.* 2004; **361**: 258–261.

42. Wayne PM, Hammerschlag R, Langevin HM, Napadow V, Park JJ, Schnyer RN. Resolving paradoxes in acupuncture research: a roundtable discussion. *J Altern Complement Med* 2009; **15**: 1039–1044.

43. Tunis SR, Stryer DB, Clancy CM. Practical clinical trials: increasing the value of clinical research for decision making in clinical and health policy. *JAMA* 2003; **290**: 1624–1632.

44. Thomas KJ, MacPherson H, Ratcliffe J, *et al.* Longer term clinical and economic benefits of offering acupuncture care to patients with chronic low back pain. *Health Technol Assess* 2005; **9**: iii–iv, ix–x, 1–109.

45. Witt CM, Jena S, Selim D, *et al.* Pragmatic randomized trial evaluating the clinical and economic effectiveness of acupuncture for chronic low back pain. *Am J Epidemiol* 2006; **164**: 487–496.

46. Manchikanti L. The growth of interventional pain management in the new millennium: a critical analysis of utilization in the Medicare population. *Pain Physician* 2004; **7**: 465–482.

47. Staal JB, de Bie RA, de Vet HC, Hildebrandt J, Nelemans P. Injection therapy for subacute and chronic low back pain: an updated Cochrane review. *Spine* 2009; **34**: 49–59.

48. Benyamin RM, Manchikanti L, Parr AT, *et al.* The effectiveness of lumbar interlaminar epidural injections in managing chronic low back and lower extremity pain. *Pain Physician* 2012; **15**: E363–404.

49. Manchikanti L, Buenaventura RM, Manchikanti KN, *et al.* Effectiveness of therapeutic lumbar transforaminal epidural steroid injections in managing lumbar spinal pain. *Pain Physician* 2012; **15**: E199–245.

50. Cohen SP. Epidural steroid injections for low back pain. *BMJ* 2011; **343**: d5310.

51. Hargunani R, Le Corroller T, Khashoggi K, Murphy KJ, Munk PL. Percutaneous vertebral augmentation: the status of vertebroplasty and current controversies. *Semin Musculoskel Radiol* 2011; **15**: 117–124.

52. Kallmes DF, Comstock BA, Heagerty PJ, *et al.* A randomized trial of vertebroplasty for osteoporotic spinal fractures. *N Engl J Med* 2009; **361**: 569–579.

53. Buchbinder R, Osborne RH, Ebeling PR, *et al.* A randomized trial of vertebroplasty for painful osteoporotic vertebral fractures. *N Engl J Med* 2009; **361**: 557–568.

54. Wardlaw D, Cummings SR, Van Meirhaeghe J, *et al.* Efficacy and safety of balloon kyphoplasty compared with non-surgical care for vertebral compression fracture (FREE): a randomised controlled trial. *Lancet* 2009; **373**: 1016–1024.

55. Voormolen MH, Mali WP, Lohle PN, *et al.* Percutaneous vertebroplasty compared with optimal pain medication treatment: short-term clinical outcome of patients with subacute or chronic painful osteoporotic vertebral compression fractures. The VERTOS study. *Am J Neuroradiol* 2007; **28**: 555–560.

56. Klazen CA, Lohle PN, de Vries J, *et al.* Vertebroplasty versus conservative treatment in acute osteoporotic vertebral compression fractures (Vertos II): an open-label randomised trial. *Lancet* 2010; **376**: 1085–1092.

57. National Center for Complementary and Alternative Medicine: What is CAM? Available at http://nccam.nih.gov/health/whatiscam, last accessed August 2012.

58. Witt, C.M. Efficacy, effectiveness, pragmatic trials — guidance on terminology and the advantages of pragmatic trials. *Forsch Komplementmed* 2009; **16**: 292–294.

59. Tunis SR, Stryer DB, Clancy CM. Practical clinical trials: increasing the value of clinical research for decision making in clinical and health policy. *JAMA* 2003; **290**: 1624–1632.

60. Schwartz D, Lellouch J. Explanatory and pragmatic attitudes in therapeutical trials. *J Clin Epidemiol* 2009; **62**: 499–505.

61. Ware JH, Hamel MB. Pragmatic trials — guides to better patient care? *N Engl J Med* 2011; **364**: 1685–1687.

62. Li A, Kaptchuk TJ. The case of acupuncture for chronic low back pain: when efficacy and comparative effectiveness conflict. *Spine* 2011; **36**: 181–182.

63. Ambrósio EM, Bloor K, Macpherson H. Costs and consequences of acupuncture as a treatment for chronic pain: A systematic review of economic evaluations conducted alongside randomised controlled trials. *Complement Ther Med* 2012; **20**: 364–374.

64. Brinkhaus B, Streng A. Routine reimbursement for acupuncture in Germany for chronic low back pain and osteoarthritis of the knee — a "healthy" decision? *Focus Altern Complement Ther* 2006; **11**: 286–288.

65. Savigny P, Watson P, Underwood M on behalf of the Guideline Development Group. Early management of persistent non-specific low back pain: summary of NICE guidance. *BMJ* 2009; **338**: 1441–1442.

66. Chou R, Qaseem A, Snow V, *et al.* Clinical Efficacy Assessment Subcommittee of the American College of Physicians; American College of Physicians; American Pain Society Low Back Pain Guidelines Panel. Diagnosis and treatment of low back pain: a joint clinical practice guideline from the American College of Physicians and the American Pain Society. *Ann Intern Med* 2007; **147**: 478–491.

CHAPTER 9

THE USE OF PLACEBOS
IN ACUPUNCTURE TRIALS

Dylan Evans

Pyschology Deparment, American University of Beirut
P.O. Box 11-0236 Beirut, Lebanon

Abstract

The standard way to establish the scientific credentials of a medical treatment is to show that it is more effective than a placebo. With pharmaceuticals, it is relatively easy to make a suitable placebo, but with acupuncture things are not so straightforward. A variety of placebos have been used in acupuncture trials. This paper examines the implications of the choice of placebo for (1) proper blinding, and (2) the nature of the hypothesis being tested in any given trial.

INTRODUCTION

The standard way to establish the scientific credentials of a medical treatment is to show that it is more effective than a placebo. This is done by carrying out a randomized controlled trial (RCT), in which participants are randomly allocated to receive either the experimental treatment or a placebo. The purpose of the placebo group is to account for the placebo effect, that is, therapeutic benefits caused by the belief that one is receiving an effective treatment rather than from the inherent properties of the experimental treatment. Without a placebo control group, it is not possible to know whether any therapeutic effects are due to the experimental treatment itself rather than to the patient's belief in that treatment.

EVIDENCE FOR THE PLACEBO EFFECT

Placebo control groups would be unnecessary if beliefs had no therapeutic effect. So what is the evidence for such belief effects? The answer to this question is controversial. On the one hand, many papers still cite the work of Henry Beecher, whose 1955 paper, "The powerful placebo", effectively began the modern study of the placebo effect. Beecher claimed that placebos could "produce gross physical change", including "objective changes at the end organ which may exceed those attributable to potent pharmacological action".[1]

On the other hand, two Danish researchers, Asbjorn Hrobjartsson and Peter Gotzsche have cast doubt on Beecher's sweeping claims.[2] Their 2001 meta-analysis of 114 trials that included both a placebo control group and a no-treatment group found that these studies fell into two distinct groups. Some had reported their results in binary terms (such as positive versus negative result) while others had used a continuous scale (such as the amount of pain relief). For the binary group, there was a small placebo effect, but the result was not significant by the normal standards of statistical research. For the studies using continuous measures, however, there was a significant beneficial placebo effect.

One problem with this study is the large range of medical problems covered by the 114 studies. In total, forty clinical conditions were examined, from asthma and smoking to menopause, marital discord and schizophrenia. Hrobjartsson and Gotzsche averaged over all these studies and, because there were relatively few studies in this sample that provided evidence in favour of the placebo effect, the negative view prevailed. But if you did the same thing for virtually any powerful drug, the result would be the same. This is because any kind of therapy that works — be it a drug, a surgical intervention, or behavioural therapy — will help people with some conditions and not others. There is no such thing as a universal remedy, a real-life cure-all, a panacea.

This, at least was the upshot of their brief conclusion. In the small print, however, they were forced to concede that for some conditions, there were noticeable placebo effects. For some conditions such as anxiety the results were too variable to allow a simple interpretation. For all sorts of pain, however, there was clear positive evidence of a significant placebo effect. Headaches, postoperative pain, and sore knees could all be relieved by a sugar pill. There was, then, some reason to suspect that, in pooling the results of studies involving so many different kinds of medical condition, the true profile of the placebo response was obscured.

Rather than asking whether or not the placebo effect exists in general, rather, we should ask which particular conditions placebos work for. Hrobjartsson and Gotzsche concede that placebos can provide effective relief from all sorts of pain. They deny that there is any good evidence that placebos work for any other symptom or condition. This conclusion does not do justice, however, to some of the studies cited. For example, two of the studies that Hrobjartsson and Gotzsche cite as providing good evidence for a placebo effect in pain relief also provide equally good evidence for a placebo effect in reducing swelling. Other studies show that stomach-ulcers, depression, and anxiety are also placebo-responsive.[3]

PLACEBO ACUPUNCTURE AND BLINDING

It is interesting to note that the few clinical trials that have found acupuncture to be better than a placebo all involve conditions known to be placebo-responsive. Trials of acupuncture for postoperative sickness and for easing neck and dental pain, for example, have found real acupuncture to outperform the sham version. When it comes to conditions that are not known to be placebo responsive, such as recovery from stroke and osteoarthritis, however, no difference has been found between acupuncture and placebo.[4] The most obvious explanation for this pattern is that blinding is not perfect in trials of acupuncture, which allows the placebo response to be activated more intensely by real acupuncture than by the sham version.

To refute this conclusion, acupuncture practitioners would need to ensure that future trials are properly blinded. This means that neither the participants nor those administering the treatment are able to tell whether the treatment is genuine acupuncture or not. This requires finding an appropriate placebo; a treatment that lacks the therapeutic ingredients specific to genuine acupuncture (if there are any) while resembling acupuncture in all other respects. With pharmaceuticals, it is relatively easy to make a suitable placebo, but with acupuncture things are not so straightforward. Clearly, a sugar pill would not constitute a good placebo for testing acupuncture, as patients would know immediately who was getting the placebo and who was getting the experimental treatment.

Some of the most rigorous trials of acupuncture have used, as a placebo, a 'sham' acupuncture treatment, in which needles are inserted into the skin just as in proper acupuncture, but not at the points corresponding to the meridians. However, the person who carries out the sham acupuncture is typically a trained acupuncturist, who knows where the meridians are supposed to lie. Such studies are not, therefore, double-blind, since the acupuncturist knows who is getting the experimental treatment and who is getting the placebo. The patients are likely to pick up on this, since doctors tend to give out subtle nonverbal cues that allow their patients to pick up on the doctor's degree of confidence in a treatment.[5] There is, therefore, no such thing as a single-blind study, where the doctor knows who is getting the placebo but the patient does not. As soon as the doctor knows, the patient does too — even if they might not be able to verbalize that knowledge. Trials are either double-blinded or not blinded at all.

ACUPUNCTURE TRIALS AND THE DUHEM-QUINE PROBLEM

The choice of placebo in acupuncture trials also raises questions about the nature of the hypothesis being tested. Acupuncture as currently practiced is a complex body of theory and practice consisting of a variety of inter-linked hypotheses and background assumptions. The needling technique of acupuncture, for example, is often (though not always) taught alongside the theories of traditional Chinese medicine, according to which a special kind of energy known as *qi* flows along channels known as meridians. If a set of trials suggests that acupuncture is no better than a placebo, then strictly speaking all that has been shown is that at least one of the hypotheses and/or background assumptions is incorrect. Yet it is never clear which hypothesis or assumption is the problem. If acupuncture is no better than sham acupuncture, for example, one possible explanation is that acupuncturists have not accurately mapped the meridians that run throughout the body.

This is an instance of what philosopher's call the Duhem-Quine problem, after Pierre Duhem and Willard Van Orman Quine. Stated in general terms, the idea is that it is impossible to test a scientific hypothesis in isolation, because an empirical test of the hypothesis requires one or more background assumptions. When the experiment does not produce the results we expect, therefore, we know that at least one of these beliefs is false, but the experiment itself does not tell us precisely which belief that is.

In sum, the scientist can never subject an isolated hypothesis to experimental test, but only a whole group of hypotheses; when the experiment is in disagreement with his predictions, what he learns is that at least one of the hypotheses constituting this group is unacceptable and ought to be modified; but the experiment does not designate which one should be changed.[6]

More formally, we can represent the logical structure of a scientific experiment as an argument with various premises and a conclusion. The principal hypothesis being tested constitutes one of the premises, but it is impossible to derive any significant conclusion from a single premise, so we must introduce other background assumptions:

(1) Principal hypothesis
(2) Background assumption 1
(3) Background assumption 2
(4) …..

Therefore: Predicted phenomenon

If we conduct the experiment and do not observe the predicted phenomenon, then we may infer by *modus tollens* that one of the assumptions (1, 2, 3, …) is not correct, but we cannot deduce which assumption that is.

Sometimes, scientists may explain a negative result by rejecting one of the background assumptions rather than the principal hypothesis. To cite a classic example, when Newton's celestial mechanics failed to correctly predict the orbit of Uranus, scientists did not conclude that Newton was wrong, but instead rejected the background assumption that the solar system contained only seven planets. This turned out to be a good move, for by calculating the location of a hypothetical eighth planet influencing the orbit of Uranus, astronomers discovered Neptune.

The same strategy is in principle open to proponents of acupuncture when confronted by studies that show acupuncture to be no better than a placebo. The nature of the particular placebo used in the trial is critically important here. If, for example, the placebo consists of inserting needles into the skin just as in proper acupuncture, but not at the points corresponding to the meridians, then the logical structure of this experiment can be represented as follows:

(1) Principal hypothesis: Acupuncture is a more effective remedy for back pain than a placebo
(2) Background assumption 1: Acupuncture works by inserting needles into the skin.
(3) Background assumption 2: The needles must be placed at particular points corresponding to the meridians.
(4) Background assumption 3: Acupuncturists have mapped the meridians accurately.
(5) Background assumption 4: The participants in this arm of the trial are suffering from back pain.
(6) Background assumption 5: The participants in this arm of the trial will be treated with genuine acupuncture.
(7) ....

Therefore: The participants in this arm of the trial will experience more relief from their back pain than those in the placebo arm of the trial.

If the predicted result is not observed, it follows that at least one of the premises is false, but we do not know for sure which premise(s) we must reject. We may choose to reject the principal hypothesis, and conclude that acupuncture is no more effective for treating back pain than a placebo. But, as with the strange orbit of Uranus, we may also explain such a negative result by rejecting one of the background assumptions rather than the principal hypothesis. We may protect the principal hypothesis from refutation by, for example, rejecting premise 4 (background assumption 3) and inferring that acupuncturists have not yet accurately mapped the meridians that run throughout the body.

A similar argument applies if a different placebo is used, but the particular conclusions will be different. Take, for example, the Park Sham Device developed by Dong Bang Acuprime. When the acupuncturist presses down on one of these sham needles, it slides inside its handle, giving the appearance of penetration but without actually penetrating the skin. Doubts have been raised about whether these devices ensure proper blinding, but that is not what interests me here. The point I wish to make is that, even if blinding is perfect, a trial in which these devices are used as the placebo does not test acupuncture per se, but the background assumption (premise 2 in the argument above) that acupuncture works by inserting needles into the skin. If the participants in the experimental arm of the trial do not experience more relief from their back pain than those in the placebo arm of the trial, we may conclude that acupuncture is no more effective for treating back pain than a placebo. Alternatively, we might conclude that acupuncture works simply by placing the needles in the correct places, and actually penetrating the skin is not essential.

Duhem's own solution to the methodological problem he identified was to appeal to the 'good sense' of scientists. But this optimistic proposal simply begs the question, for in the controversial cases where the Duhem-Quine problem is most pressing, scientists who draw very different conclusions are all convinced that is they who have good sense and others who lack it.

CONCLUSION

In conclusion, the role of placebos in clinical trials of acupuncture raises two important problems. First, the difficulty of constructing a placebo that could ensure double blinding in acupuncture trials means that when such trials show acupuncture to be more effective than the placebo, the most obvious explanation is that the placebo response to be activated more intensely by real acupuncture than by the sham version. The result is that acupuncture seems better than a placebo only when the condition being treated is, in fact, placebo responsive. This should worry acupuncture practitioners, since it suggests that acupuncture may be a pure placebo.[3]

Second, the choice of placebo will also depend on one's theory about how acupuncture is supposed to work. If this theory specifies the needles must be placed accurately at various points on various meridians, then the Park Sham Device may be appropriate, but if this theory specifies that the skin must be penetrated, then this device will not be suitable. Of course, it may be that these details have not been made sufficiently explicit by the proponents of acupuncture, in which case the debate about suitable placebos for use in acupuncture trials might provide a useful opportunity for acupuncturists to develop their theories in more detail.

Or perhaps they could abandon their theories altogether, and focus on specifying more precisely the details of the technique. This may actually be a more fruitful path, since it is the association of acupuncture with dubious theories about *qi* and meridians that is largely responsible for the general skepticism with which acupuncture is viewed by mainstream medicine. If the techniques of acupuncture could be separated from the dubious theories that sometimes accompany them, the way would be open to a much more profound dialog between acupuncture and mainstream medicine.

REFERENCES

1. Beecher HK, The powerful placebo *J Am Med Assoc* 1955; **159**: 1602.
2. Hrobjartsson H and Gotzsche PC, Is the placebo powerless? — An analysis of clinical trials comparing placebo with no treatment *New Eng J Med* 2001; **344**: 1594.
3. Evans D, *Placebo: The Belief Effect*. London: HarperCollins, 2003.
4. BMA, *Acupuncture: Efficacy, Safety and Practice*. London: Harwood, 2000.
5. Gracely RH *et al.* Clinicians' expectations influence placebo analgesia. *Lancet* 1985; **1**: 43.
6. Duhem P, *The Aim and Structure of Physical Theory*, trans. from 2nd ed. by Wiener PM; (originally published as *La Théorie Physique: Son Objet et sa Structure*. Paris: Marcel Riviera & Cie. 1914), Princeton, NJ: Princeton University Press, 1954.

CHAPTER 10

IMPROVING THE QUALITY OF RANDOMIZED CONTROLLED TRIALS (RCTS) IN ACUPUNCTURE

Zhaoxiang Bian, Chungwah Cheng,
Linda Chan, Mandy Cheung and Min Li
School of Chinese Medicine
Hong Kong Baptist University, HKSAR

Zhixiu Lin
School of Chinese Medicine
The Chinese University of Hong Kong, HKSAR

Abstract

In order to evaluate the clinical efficacy of acupuncture, the use of randomization controlled trial (RCT) for acupuncture is increasing rapidly recently, with different control groups. The objective of this paper are: (1) To systemically review the quality of reporting of RCTs with acupuncture; and (2) to discuss the design of sham acupuncture and its existing problem. Methodology: A search of the OVID and EMBASE database was conducted to identify the articles of RCTs with acupuncture for the low back pain. A revised CONSORT checklist and STRICTA checklist, containing 78 items with 23 items specifically for acupuncture, was applied as an assessment instrument to assess the quality of the reporting. Result: There are 44 articles of RCTs of acupuncture which were met our requirement. The overall reporting quality of the RCTs of acupuncture which was assessed with the revised

CONSORT checklist and STRICTA checklist varied between 19% and 70%, with a median score of 43% (standard deviation 12%). As for sham acupuncture, there are four types of design mainly. They are superficial needling on acupuncture point, non-specific needling control, non-insertive simulated needling control and transcutaneous electrical nerve stimulation (TENS). Conclusion: The overall reporting quality of RCTs of acupuncture is low. It is necessary to improve the reporting quality. The control design of acupuncture should be improved too.

INTRODUCTION

The purpose of clinical trial with Chinese Medicine is to evaluate the safety and efficacy of Chinese Medicine, while the evaluation of efficacy is based on the control between the tested intervention and the control group(s). If there is no control, it is difficult to evaluate the efficacy of an intervention. Therefore, to set up a control in a trial is very important for the evaluation of efficacy of an intervention.

In the last decades, in order to evaluate the efficacy of acupuncture, randomization controlled trials (RCT) were designed and conducted. In those trials, different type of controls has been applied. But there are no much studies to evaluate the quality of those reporting, especially for the control designs. The aim of our research is to (1) systemically review and analyze the quality of reporting paper of RCT with acupuncture; (2) discuss the existing problem of design of sham acupuncture; (3) evaluate the advantage and disadvantage of different type of design of sham acupuncture; and (4) provide suggestions for improving the design of sham design.

MATERIALS AND METHOD

Search Strategy

The papers which are related to the RCT with sham acupuncture in low back pain can be identified from the Ovid MEDLINE(R), Ovid OLDMEDLINE(R) and EMBASE database. The following search strategy was used:

Step. 1   exp acupuncture therapy/ or exp electroacupuncture/ or exp acupuncture/ (26279)
Step. 2   (acupunctur$ or Electroacupunctur$ or Electro-acupunctur$). tw. (20823)

Step. 3   or/1–2 (28920)

Step. 4   exp acupressure/ or exp acupuncture, ear/ or exp moxibustion/ (15573)

Step. 5   (auriculoacupuncture or acupressure or moxibustion).tw. (1773)

Step. 6   exp meridians/ or exp acupuncture points/ (16665)

Step. 7   or/4–6 (17950)

Step. 8   3 not 7 (11293)

Step. 9   randomized controlled trial$.pt. (264806)

Step. 10   exp randomized controlled trial$/ (433439)

Step. 11   Randomized Controlled Trial$.tw. (51175)

Step. 12   exp random allocation/ (89718)

Step. 13   random allocation.tw. (1508)

Step. 14   exp double blind method/ (175236)

Step. 15   exp single blind method/ (20557)

Step. 16   ((singl$ or doubl$ or trebl$ or tripl$) adj (blind$ or mask$)).tw. (202497)

Step. 17   exp PLACEBOS/ or exp placebo/ (168514)

Step. 18   exp sham treatment/ or exp sham procedure/ (28196)

Step. 19   (placebo$ or sham treatment or sham procedure).tw. (238038)

Step. 20   exp controlled clinical trial/ (257705)

Step. 21   controlled clinical trial.pt. (78327)

Step. 22   ((controlled adj3 trial?) or (controlled adj3 stud$)).tw. (254313)

Step. 23   or/9–22 (905061)

Step. 24   8 and 23 (1768)

Step. 25   (note or comment or comment editorial or bibliography or commentary or editorial or letter).pt. (1901756)

Step. 26   (review or systematic review or meta analysis).pt. (2378919)

Step. 27   practice guideline$.pt. (12924)

Step. 28   or/25–27 (4266366)

Step. 29   exp Low Back Pain/ (30198)

Step. 30   exp Low Back Pain/ (30198)

Step. 31   (low back pain$ or low back$ache$ or Lumbago or Lumbal$ or Lumbar or Ischialgia or Intervertebral Disk).tw. (138802)

Step. 32   or/29–31 (148439)

Step. 33   24 and 32 (132)

Step. 34   33 not 28 (94)

Step. 35   remove duplicates from 34 (89)

Step. 36   limit 35 to human (77)
Step. 37   from 36 keep 1–77 (77)

After a search with the above strategy, a list of 77 papers was found. Among the 77 papers, the following exclusion criteria were used to sort out the finalized list of paper for analysis. Exclusion criteria:

(1) The paper is related to an animal study or experiment.
(2) The paper is not related to acupuncture.
(3) The paper is not related to low back pain.
(4) The paper is not related to a placebo-controlled trial.
(5) The paper is not related to clinical study.
(6) The paper is written in Germany.
(7) Full paper cannot be found.

After sorting out the paper with the above exclusion criteria, there are a total of 44 papers which are related to our research. The papers were downloaded from the electronic resource database of libraries of Hong Kong Baptist University, The Chinese University of Hong Kong and Hong Kong University. For those papers which cannot be downloaded from the electronic resource database, hardcopies were collected from the universities instead. Therefore, these 44 papers were selected to analyze for our research.[1–44]

Assessment of Quality of Trials

Acupuncture treatment and control group interventions in parallel-group randomized trials of acupuncture are not always precisely reported. In an attempt to improve standards, an international group of experienced acupuncturists and researchers devised a set of recommendations, designating them STRICTA (Table 1): STandards for Reporting Interventions in Controlled Trials of Acupuncture. Thus, STRICTA checklist is specially designed for acupuncture and it consists of five aspects to evaluate the reporting of acupuncture, including the rationale of acupuncture trial, needling details, treatment regimen, cointerventions, and practitioner background and control intervention. STRICTA checklist is then added

Table 1. STRICTA checklist.

Intervention	Item	Description
Acupuncture	1	Style of acupuncture Rationale for treatment (e.g., syndrome patterns, segmental levels, trigger points) and individualization if used Literature sources to justify rationale
Needling details	2	Points used (unilateral/bilateral) Numbers of needles inserted Depths of insertion (e.g., cun or tissue level) Responses elicited (e.g., *de qi* or twitch response) Needle stimulation (e.g., manual or electrical) Needle retention time Needle type (gauge, length, and manufacturer or material)
Treatment regimen	3	Number of treatment sessions Frequency of treatment
Cointerventions	4	Other interventions (e.g., moxibustion, cupping, herbs, exercises, lifestyle advice)
Practitioner	5	Duration of relevant training Background length of clinical experience Expertise in specific condition
Control Intervention(s)	6	Intended effect of control intervention and its appropriateness to research question and, if appropriate, blinding of participants (e.g. active comparison, minimally active, penetrating or non-penetrating sham, inert) Explanations given to patients of treatment and control interventions, details of control intervention (precise description, as for Item 2 above, and other items if different) Sources that justify choice of control

into the CONSORT (Consolidated Standards for Reporting Trials), acting as an extension of the CONSORT guidelines for the specific requirements of acupuncture studies which is named as revised CONSORT checklist and STRICTA checklist (Table 2).

Table 2.   Revised CONSORT checklist and STRICTA checklist.

SECTION /Topic	Old #	New #	Description
TITLE	1	1	Identifies study as a RCT
ABSTRACT		2	Has an abstract
		3	Has a structured format
		4	Gives hypothesis (or rationale)
		5	Gives number of patients
		6	States whether analysis was by intention-to-treat
		7	Gives method of randomization
		8	States results
INTRODUCTION	2	9	Scientific background
		10	Explanation of rationale
METHODS	3	11	Diagnostic criteria
		12	Inclusion criteria
		13	Exclusion criteria
		14	Informed consent form
		15	Ethic committee approval
		16	Settings and locations where the data were collected
Intervention	STRICTA	17	Style of acupuncture (Traditional Chinese Medicine or western Medicine)
		18	Syndrome patterns
		19	Segmental levels
		20	Trigger points
		21	Individualization, if any
		22	Literature sources to justify rationale

(*Continued*)

Table 2. (*Continued*).

SECTION /Topic	Old #	New #	Description
		23	Points used (unilateral/bilateral)
		24	Numbers of needles inserted
		25	Depths of insertion (e.g., cun or tissue level)
		26	Responses elicited (e.g., *de qi* or twitch response)
		27	Needle stimulation (e.g., manual or electrical)
		28	Needle retention time
		29	Needle type (gauge, length, and manufacturer or material)
		30	Number of treatment sessions
		31	Frequency of treatment
		32	Other interventions (e.g., moxibustion, cupping, herbs, exercises, lifestyle advice)
		33	Duration of relevant training
		34	Length of clinical experience
		35	Expertise in specific condition
		36	Intended effect of control intervention and its appropriateness to research question
		37	Explanations given to patients of treatment
		38	Control interventions
		39	Details of control intervention (precise description, as for Item 2 above, and other items if different)
		40	Sources that justify choice of control
Objectives	5	41	Specific objectives
		42	Hypothesis
Outcomes	6	43	Defined primary outcome measures
		44	Defined secondary outcome measures
		45	Methods to enhance the quality of outcomes measurements

(*Continued*)

Table 2. *(Continued)*.

SECTION /Topic	Old #	New #	Description
Sample size	7	46	Sample size
		47	States sample size calculation
		48	Explanation of any interim analyses
		49	Explanation of stopping rules
Randomization			
Sequence generation	8	50	State method to generate the random allocation sequence
		51	States whether sequence was concealed until interventions were assigned
Randomization Allocation concealment	9	52	States method to implement the random allocation sequence
Randomization			
Implementation	10	53	States that generated the allocation sequence
		54	Who enrolled participants
		55	Who assigned participants to their groups
Blinding	11	56	States that the trial is blinded or open.
		57	Participants were blinded to group assignment
		58	Investigators were blinded to group assignment
		59	Assessors were blinded to group assignment
		60	States how the success of blinding was evaluated
Statistical methods	12	61	Defines statistical methods
RESULTS			
Participant flow	13	62	Flow of participants through each stage
		63	Describes protocol deviations and reasons
Recruitment	14	64	Dates defined periods of recruitment

(Continued)

Table 2. (*Continued*)

SECTION /Topic	Old #	New #	Description
Baseline data	15	65	Baseline of clinical characteristics of each group
Numbers analyzed	16	66	Actual number of participants in each group
		67	"Intention-to-treat" analysis
		68	States withdrawal/dropout
Outcomes and estimation	17	69	Summary of results for each group with primary and secondary outcomes
		70	Estimates effect size
		71	Estimates precision of effect size (95% confidence interval)
Ancillary analyses	18	72	Addresses multiplicity by reporting any other analyses performed including subgroup analyses and adjusted analyses
Adverse events	19	73	States important adverse events or side effects
DISCUSSION			
Interpretation	20	74	Interpretation of results / states dangers associated with multiplicity of analyses and outcomes
		75	Interpretation of the results / states sources of potential bias
Generalizability	21	76	Generalizability (external validity) of the trial findings
Overall evidence	22	77	Interpretation of results in context of current evidence
		78	Total / mean

Data Extraction and Analysis

The assessment of quality of RCT of each paper with revised CONSORT checklist and STRICTA checklist was carried by two reviewers independently (Ka-Lin Chan and Wai-Man Cheung). If discrepancy due to inappropriate data extraction appeared after the two individual assessments, all disagreements were then resolved by achieving consensus involving a third reviewer (Zhao-Xiang Bian). After achieved the final consensus in the assessment, the data was then processed in Microsoft Excel for further analysis.

RESULTS

Literature Search

There are 44 articles of RCTs of acupuncture which were included in this review. The majority of papers (33 articles, 75%) were published after 2000 and only the minority of papers (11 articles, 25%) was published between 1980 and 1999. In addition, 40 articles were published in English while four articles were published in Chinese.

Reporting Quality

The total number of RCTs reported for each item in the checklist was calculated and shown in the Tables 3 and 4. The summary of scores for each item varied between 0% to 100%, with a mean of 16.68. Table 3 provides a summary of reporting rate for each item in the checklist. The overall reporting quality of the RCTs of acupuncture, based on the revised CONSORT checklist and STRICTA checklist, varied between 19% and 70%, with a median score of 43% (standard deviation 12%). Table 4 provides a summary of overall reporting quality for each RCT article included in this review.

Title and abstract

Among 44 papers, only 18 (41%) papers identified their studies as RCT in the title. And 43 (98%) papers have an abstract while only 29 (66%) papers with a structured format. Only one (3%) papers gave hypothesis (or rationale) in the abstract. Forty-two (95%) papers stated numbers of patients in the abstract. Only two (5%) papers stated whether analysis was by intention-to-treat and none of paper state method of randomization. There were 43 (98%) papers with clear presentation of results in the abstract.

Table 3. Revised CONSORT and STRICTA checklist and with results.

SECTION/Topic	Old #	New #	Description	N	%
TITLE	1	1	Identifies study as a RCT	18	41
ABSTRACT		2	Has an abstract	43	98
		3	Has a structured format	29	66
		4	Gives hypothesis (or rationale)	1	2
		5	Gives number of patients	42	95
		6	States whether analysis was by intention-to-treat	2	5
		7	Gives method of randomization	0	0
		8	States results	43	98
INTRODUCTION	2	9	Scientific background	36	82
		10	Explanation of rationale	7	16
METHODS	3	11	Diagnostic criteria	5	11
		12	Inclusion criteria	30	68
		13	Exclusion criteria	33	75
		14	Informed consent form	32	73
		15	Ethic committee approval	21	48
		16	Settings and locations where the data were collected	30	68
Intervention	STRICTA	17	Style of acupuncture (Traditional Chinese Medicine or Western Medicine)	39	89
		19	Syndrome patterns	3	7
		20	Segmental levels	1	2
		21	Trigger points	30	68
		22	Individualization, if any	17	39

(Continued)

Table 3. (*Continued*).

SECTION/Topic	Old #	New #	Description	N	%
		23	Literature sources to justify rationale	11	25
		24	Points used (unilateral/ bilateral)	6	14
		25	Numbers of needles inserted	8	18
		26	Depths of insertion (e.g., cun or tissue level)	24	55
		27	Responses elicited (e.g., *de qi* or twitch response)	27	61
		28	Needle stimulation (e.g., manual or electrical)	18	41
		29	Needle retention time	37	84
		30	Needle type (gauge, length, and manufacturer or material)	29	66
		31	Number of treatment sessions	39	89
		32	Frequency of treatment	30	68
		33	Other interventions (e.g., moxibustion, cupping,herbs, exercises, lifestyle advice)	10	23
		34	Duration of relevant training	2	5
		35	Length of clinical experience	21	48
		36	Expertise in specific condition	14	32
		37	Intended effect of control intervention and its appropriateness to research question	44	100

(*Continued*)

Table 3. (*Continued*)

SECTION/Topic	Old #	New #	Description	N	%
		38	Explanations given to patients of treatment	8	18
		39	Control interventions	39	89
		40	Details of control intervention (precise description, as for Item 2 above, and other items if different)	2	5
		41	Sources that justify choice of control	7	16
Objectives	5	42	Specific objectives	35	80
		43	Hypothesis	3	7
Outcomes	6	44	Defined primary outcome measures	14	32
		45	Defined secondary outcome measures	12	27
		46	Methods to enhance the quality of outcomes measurements	0	0
Sample size	7	47	Sample size	Average 402	
		48	States sample size calculation	9	20
		49	Explanation of any interim analyses	10	23
		50	Explanation of stopping rules	2	5
Randomization					
Sequence generation	8	51	State method to generate the random allocation sequence	9	20
		52	States whether sequence was concealed until interventions were assigned	10	28

(*Continued*)

Table 3.   (*Continued*)

SECTION/Topic	Old #	New #	Description	N	%
Randomization					
Allocation concealment	9	53	States method to implement the random allocation sequence	11	25
Randomization					
Implementation	10	54	States that generated the allocation sequence	3	7
		55	Who enrolled participants	0	0
		56	Who assigned participants to their groups	4	9
Blinding	11	57	States that the trial is blinded or open.	9	20
		58	Participants were blinded to group assignment	15	34
		59	Investigators were blinded to group assignment	5	11
		60	Assessors were blinded to group assignment	14	32
		61	States how the success of blinding was evaluated	2	5
Statistical methods	12	62	Defines statistical methods	37	84
RESULTS					
Participant flow	13	63	Flow of participants through each stage	22	50
		64	Describes protocol deviations and reasons	12	27

(*Continued*)

Table 3. (*Continued*)

SECTION/Topic	Old #	New #	Description	N	%
Recruitment	14	65	Dates defined periods of recruitment	13	30
Baseline data	15	66	Baseline of clinical characteristics of each group	27	61
Numbers analyzed	16	67	Actual number of participants in each group	34	77
		68	'Intention-to-treat' analysis	10	23
		69	States withdrawal/ dropout	21	48
Outcomes and estimation	17	70	Summary of results for each group with primary and secondary outcomes	31	70
		71	Estimates effect size	5	11
		72	Estimates precision of effect size (95% confidence interval)	5	11
Ancillary analyses	18	73	Addresses multiplicity by reporting any other analyses performed including subgroup analyses and adjusted analyses	1	2
Adverse events	19	74	States important adverse events or side effects	15	34
DISCUSSION					
Interpretation	20	75	Interpretation of results/ states dangers associated with multiplicity of analyses and outcomes	1	2
		76	Interpretation of the results/states sources of potential bias	9	20

(*Continued*)

Table 3. (*Continued*)

SECTION/Topic	Old #	New #	Description	N	%
Generalizability	21	77	Generalizability (external validity) of the trial findings	0	0
Overall evidence	22	78	Interpretation of results in context of current evidence	33	75
		79	Total/mean	16.86	

N = Number of RCTs reported certain item (%).

Table 4. Summary of overall reporting quality of RCTs of acupuncture.

Author	Year Published	Items reported	Score (%)	Author	Year Published	Items reported	Score (%)
S. Kenned	2008	41	53	Yeung CKN	2003	41	53
Rtensson LM	2008	41	53	Giles LGF	2003	39	51
Zhuang Zq	2008	25	32	Tsukayama H	2002	34	44
Wong	2007	24	31	Molsberger AF	2002	49	64
Haake M	2007	51	66	Ceccherelli F	2002	33	43
Wu YC	2007	35	45	Leibing E	2002	47	61
Linde K	2007	27	35	Carlsson CPO	2001	43	56
Harbach H	2007	32	42	Kalauokalani D	2001	27	35
Zhou YL	2006	29	38	Wedenberg K	2000	25	32
Thomas KJ	2006	37	48	Wang RR	2000	30	39
Ratcliff J	2006	30	39	Giles LGF	1999	31	40
Witt CM	2006	31	40	MacPherson H	1999	23	30
Huang SR	2006	33	43	Thomas M	1994	27	35
Lund I	2006	36	47	Kitade T	1990	20	26
Brinkhaus B	2006	41	53	The practitioner	1988	15	19
Thomas KJ	2005	54	70	Lehmann TR	1986	25	32
Tsui MLK	2004	34	44	Martelete M	1985	19	25

(*Continued*)

Table 4. (*Continued*).

Author	Year Published	Items reported	Score (%)	Author	Year Published	Items reported	Score (%)
Silva JBGD	2004	33	43	Lehmann TR	1983	19	25
Kvorning N	2004	35	45	Macdonald AJR	1983	28	36
Chu J	2004	27	35	Mendelson G	1983	35	45
Meng CF	2003	45	58	Coan RM	1980	17	22
Kerr DP	2003	36	47	Gunn CC	1980	28	36
				Mean		33	43

Introduction

There were 36 (82%) articles that provided scientific background while only seven (16%) articles included an explanation of rationale about the RCT studied.

Objectives

There were only 35 (80%) studies that stated their specific objectives and only three (7%) studies that stated their hypothesis in their reports.

Methods-Participants

Not all papers stated the diagnostic criteria of disease clearly. Only five (11%) papers provided diagnostic criteria. Thirty (68%) papers gave inclusion criteria while 33 (75%) papers gave exclusion criteria. In addition, 32 (73%) papers stated informed consent form and 21 (48%) papers stated the RCT has been approval by ethic committee. Only 30 (68%) papers gave information about the settings and locations where the data were collected.

Methods-Intervention

There were 39 (89%) papers that stated the style of acupuncture (Traditional Chinese Medicine or Western Medicine) chosen for intervention in the trial. Only three (7%) paper reported syndrome patterns of disease and only one (2%) papers reported segmental levels. Only 30 (68%) papers stated clearly the acupoints used and only 17 (39%) papers reported if any individualization were applied in the study. Only 11 articles provided literature sources to justify rationale of acupoint selection, while six (14%) papers reported that the points used unilaterally or bilaterally. Further, only eight (18%) papers gave the numbers of needles inserted, and only 24 (55%) papers stated the depth of insertion (e.g. cun or tissue level). Around half of articles reported the following items: 27 (62%) papers stated responses elicited (e.g., *de qi* or twitch response); 18 (41%) papers stated needle stimulation (e.g., manual or electrical); 37 (84%) papers stated needle retention time; 29 (66%) papers reported needle type (gauge, length, and manufacturer or material); 39 (89%) papers reported number of treatment sessions; and 30 (68%) papers reported frequency of treatment. For other interventions such as moxibustion, cupping, herbs, exercises, lifestyle advice, only ten studies reported in the trial. For information related to the background of interventionist, only two (5%) papers provided the duration of relevant training, 21 (48%) papers provided length of clinical experience and 14 (32%) papers stated expertise in specific condition. All 44 articles stated the intended effect of control intervention and its appropriateness to research question. Only eight (18%) study provided explanations to patients regarding treatment. There are 39 (89%) papers reported the control intervention in brief, while two (5%) papers stated details of control intervention. Only seven papers reported the sources that justify choice of control.

Sample Size, Randomization, Blinding and Statistical Methods

The average sample sized was 402. All 44 papers stated sample size and only nine (20%) papers stated sample size calculation in the study. Only ten (23%) papers gave explanation of any interim analyses while only two (%) papers gave explanation of stopping rules of trials. For the method of generation of the random allocation sequence, it was provided by only nine (20%) articles. Only ten (23%) articles stated whether sequence was allocation concealment. For the method of implement of the random allocation sequence, it was only stated by 11 (25%) papers. For the randomization implementation, only three (7%) papers stated who generated the allocation sequence but none of paper stated who enrolled participants. Only four (7%) papers stated who assigned participants to the corresponding groups. For blinding, only nine (20%) studies stated that the trial was blinded or open; 15 (34%) studies reported that participants were blinded to group assignment; five (11%) studies reported that investigators were blinded to group assignment; and 14 (32%) studies reported that assessors were blinded to group assignment. Only two (4%) studies stated how the success of blinding was evaluated. For statistical methods, 37 (84%) studies defined statistical methods.

Results and Outcomes

Half of articles (50%) provided the flow of participants through each stage. Twelve (27%) papers described protocol deviations and reasons, and 13 (30%) papers reported dates defined periods of recruitment. The baseline of clinical characteristics of each group was reported by 27 (61%) papers. For numbers of participants analyzed in the results, 34 (77%) papers stated the actual number of participants in each group, and ten (23%) papers stated with "intention-to-treat" analysis, and 21 (48%) papers stated withdrawal or dropout.

The definition of primary outcome measures was provided by 14 (32%) articles only while the definition of secondary outcome measures was only provided by 12 (27%) papers. None of study studied the methods to enhance the quality of outcomes measurements. There are 31 (70%) papers that reported the summary of results for each group with primary and secondary outcomes. Only five (11%) papers stated the estimation of effect size while only five (11%) papers stated the estimation precision of effect size (95% confidence interval). For the multiplicity by reporting any other analyses performed including subgroup analyses and adjusted analyses, it was addressed by one (2%) paper only. There were 15 (34%) papers that stated important adverse events or side effects.

Discussion

The dangers associated with multiplicity of analyses and outcomes were only stated by one (2%) paper and nine (20%) papers reported the sources of potential bias. None of paper stated the generalizability (external validity) of the trial findings and 33 (75%) papers stated the interpretation of results in context of current evidence.

DESIGN OF CONTROL GROUP

Among 44 trials, 39 RCTs has the set-up of control group, with four main types including superficial needling on acupuncture point (one trial), non-specific needling control (ten trials), non-insertive simulated needling control (one trial), mock transcutaneous electrical nerve stimulation (TENS) (four trials) and other type of control such as no treatment control and normal care control (23 trials).

Type 1: Superficial Needling on Acupuncture Point

A shorter or thinner needle, comparing with that in the treatment group, is inserted subcutaneously over the acupuncture point, with depth of insertion of 1–2 mm. No manipulation of needle like rotation, lifting and thrusting is applied. In this type of control, no 'de qi' sensation, such as numbness, heaviness and soreness, can be felt by the participants, because the needle is inserted superficially without manipulation. Moreover, this type of control can only be used for the points which are not easily observed by the patient e.g. head, back. Besides, therapeutic effect due to insertion into acupuncture point may be underestimated.

Type 2: Non-Specific Location Needling Control

In this type of control, needles were inserted into locations that were believed to be ineffective for the condition being treated. No Specific requirement about the depth of insertion, either superficially (1–2mm) or deeply (10–20mm). Normally, no manual stimulation is needed.

The validity of this type of control group depends on the assumption that for a specific condition, acupuncture is effective at some anatomic sites.43 It is questionable to define the accurate position of the ineffective site as well as to prove that there is no effect for the condition being treated with the insertion of needles into location on the body.

Type 3. Non-Insert Needling Control

Non-insert needling controls have several types including cocktail sticks, acupuncture needle guidetubes (without the needle), toothpicks inserted in guidetubes and Streitberger's placebo needle, in which special non-insert needles with a retractable handle and blunt tip were used, thus to induce pricking sensation felt by the patient.43 Interestingly, some investigation found that toothpicks inserted in guidetubes were more convincing than other potential simulated needling techniques which were tested before (cocktail sticks, acupuncture needle guidetubes) and more comfortable for the acupuncturists because of the similarity with real acupuncture practice. The feel of participants towards toothpicks, cocktail sticks, acupunctures needle guidetubes (without the needle) may be different among different populations therefore, it is difficult to imitate the real acupuncture. But for acupuncture-naïve person, it will be more easily passed off as true acupuncture.

Type 4: Mock Transcutaneous Electrical Nerve Stimulation (TENS) Control

The use of non-functioning TENS (without the needles taped to the skin) is one another type of control. An electrical apparatus is connected to acupuncture point or sham point via electrodes but without any or with very low electrical impulses delivery. The patients being tested do not have any muscle stimulation. Because the patients tested do not have any sensation of electrical impulse and muscle stimulation, different sensation may be distinguished by the subjects. Further, low electrical impulse delivery may have potential therapeutic effect. In addition, mock TENS is for the control of TENS only.

DISCUSSION

Reporting of RCTs is the important way for readers to understand what have done in the trial. From the result of assessment, the quality of reporting of RCTs of acupuncture is low. The majority of papers did not report the required items adequately based on the revised CONSORT checklist and STRICTA checklist. The items suggested in the checklist are necessarily reported as detailed as possible in order to facilitate the communication between authors, peer reviewers, editors, and readers,[44,45] although the checklist may not be the best guideline for the improvement of report.[46] Therefore, the application of the revised CONSORT checklist and STRICTA checklist is necessary to ensure the reporting quality of RCTs with acupuncture. Some researchers have suggested that the quality of reporting of RCT is not indicative of the quality of its execution, and some reviewers found that bad reporting simply reflected the bad methodology and design of the trials.[47] Therefore, it is necessary to maintain the quality of reporting with high standard in order to indicate the quality of the execution of the trial.

From the results shown by the checklist, it can be found that more than half of RCTs articles do not identify their study as RCT in the title. It is necessary to identify the study as RCT in the title since it is first information received by the reader. The majority of papers contain an abstract but some of them are not written with the structured format and most papers do not include hypothesis, intention-to-treat and method of randomization which are important information for readers to understand the papers.

For the reporting of the methodology of clinical trials, most of important elements like diagnostic criteria, sample size calculation, randomization, blinding were not provided by majority of articles. The importance of reporting the methodology clearly is to provide the enough information how the trial was designed and implemented. If the methods cannot be reported clearly, it is difficulty for readers, reviewers, editors, etc., to judge how the trial has been designed and implemented. For example, the diagnostic criteria, inclusion and exclusion criteria are very important for the participants' selection. When the information cannot be reported clearly, it is impossible for readers to understand the targeted group of the trial, or cannot form a clear profile about the characteristics of participants. Similar requests for the other parts of methods in the trial, such as randomization, blinding, allocation concealment, etc. Currently, an increasing number of medical journals require the authors to report the sample size calculation process in accordance so that the reader can understand the rationale behind why the certain sample of participants are needed. Also, it has to be ensured that trials have proper sample sizes so that the differences among groups can be detected.[48]

The control design is an important part of RCT. In the RCTs of acupuncture, different types of control group can be chosen such as placebo (sham control), active control, and no treatment control groups. Ideal sham control design about acupuncture should: (1) not have any therapeutic effect; and (2) the design should be identical such that the practitioner or participants cannot detect the difference between the sham design and real acupuncture. For the four types of controls used in the trial of low back pain, the design could be improved to some extents. Since therapeutic effect may be induced by superficial needling on acupuncture point, choosing non-specific needling control or non-insert needling control probably can reduce this effect. For non-specific location needling control, more research and evidence should be provided to support the effect of these locations on the specific condition. The design of the non-insert needling control should be improved so as to make the RCT participants believe that they are receiving the real acupuncture. For mock TENS, the low electrical impulse inducing any potential therapeutic effects can be avoided for the benefit of this study. When the participants have acupuncture experience, it is very easy for them to recognize whether it is false acupuncture.

To determine the proper control design of acupuncture treatment, it is necessary to determine what the research question in the trial is, and what is the major components should be detected in the trial. All aspects in the process of acupuncture should be taken into consideration when design the control group. For example, a design with an electroacupuncture in one specific acupoint includes the following variable aspects: (1) electro-related aspects, such as power, frequency; and (2) acupoint. The control design could be targeted electro-related aspects; and/ or acupoint-related aspects. Therefore, it is necessary to take all related aspects into consideration.

LIMITATIONS

There are two limitations in our research. First, the source of articles are limited since there were only 44 articles of RCTs with acupuncture used for the reporting quality assessment with the revised CONSORT checklist and STRICTA checklist. Moreover, all 44 articles are related to low back pain only. Therefore, it could be concluded that the result from our research may not represent for all other RCTs of acupuncture. Furthermore, the checklist used in our research just provided some basic requirements for reporting. The checklist may not the only standard for assessment of the reporting quality.

CONCLUSION

The overall reporting quality of RCTs of acupuncture is low with the assessment of the revised CONSORT checklist and STRICTA checklist. The quality of reporting of RCTs of acupuncture needs to be improved by including the reporting of all items given in the checklist. The design of control with acupuncture should be improved too.

REFERENCES

1. Kennedy S, Baxter GD, Kerr DP, Bradbury I, Park J, McDonough SM. Acupuncture for acute non-specific low back pain: a pilot randomised non-penetrating sham controlled trial, *Complementary Ther Med* 2008, **16**(3): 139–146.
2. Martensson L, Stener-Victorin E, Wallin G. Acupuncture versus subcutaneous injections of sterile water as treatment for labour pain. *Acta Obstetricia et Gynecologica Scandinavica* 2008, **87**(2): 171–177.
3. Wang ZL, Chan LF, Zhu WM, Observation study of TNBS for low back pain. Chinese Acupuncture, 2007, **27**(9): 657–659.
4. Haake M, Muller H-H, Schade-Brittinger C, Basler HD, Schafer H, Maier C, Endres HG, Trampisch HJ, Molsberger A. German Acupuncture Trials (GERAC) for chronic low back pain: randomized, multicenter, blinded, parallel-group trial with 3 groups, *Arc Int Med* 2007; **167**(17): 1892–1898.

5. Wu YS, Zhang BM, Wong ZM, Zhang JF, Zhao P, Liu GZ, Electroacupuncture on HJ for the acute low back pain. *Chin Acupunct* 2007; **27**(1): 3–5.

6. Klaus L Inde, Claudia M, Witt Andrea S Treng, Wolfgang Weidenhammer, Stefan Wagenpfeil, Benno Brinkhaus, Stefan N Willich, Dieter Melchart. The impact of patient expectations on outcomes in four randomized controlled trials of acupuncture in patients with chronic pain. *Pain* 2007; **128**(3): 264–271.

7. Harbach H, Moll R-H Boedeker, Vigelius-Rauch U, Otto H, Muehling J, Hempelmann G, Markart P. Minimal immunoreactive plasma beta-endorphin and decrease of cortisol at standard analgesia or different acupuncture techniques. *Eur J Anaesthesiol*, 2007; **24**(4): 370–376.

8. Zhou YL, Zhang SJ, Su KS, Chan JF, Liu P, Liu YJ, Lin KP, Hu P. Three angle needles for low back pain. *Chin Acupunct* 2006; **26**(12): 847–850

9. Thomas KJ, MacPherson H, Thorpe L, Brazier J, Fitter M, Campbell M J, Roman M, Walters SJ and Nicholl J. Randomised controlled trial of a short course of traditional acupuncture compared with usual care for persistent non-specific low back pain. *Brit Med J* 2006; **333**(7569): 623.

10. Claudia M. Witt1, Susanne Jena1, Dagmar Selim1, Benno Brinkhaus1, Thomas Reinhold1, Katja Wruck1, Bodo Liecker2, Klaus Linde3, Karl Wegscheider4, and Stefan N. Willich1. Pragmatic randomized trial evaluating the clinical and economic effectiveness of acupuncture for chronic low back pain. *Am J Epidemiol*, 2006; **164**(5): 487–496.

11. Huang SY, Shi YY, Zhan HS. Electroacupuncture in single acupoint for low back pain: a control study. *Chin Acupunct* 2006; **26**(5): 319–321

12. Lund I, Thomas L, Lena L, Elisabeth Svensson, Decrease of pregnant women's pelvic pain after acupuncture: a randomized controlled single-blind study. *Acta Obstetricia et Gynecologica Scandinavica* 2006; **85**(1): 12–19,

13. Benno Brinkhaus, Claudia M. Witt, Susanne Jena, Klaus Linde; Andrea Streng, Stefan Wagenpfeil, Dominik Irnich, Heinz-Ulrich Walther, Dieter Melchart, Stefan N. Willich. Acupuncture in patients with chronic low back pain: a randomized controlled trial. *Arch Int Med* 2006; **166**(4): 450–457.

14. Thomas KJ, MacPherson H, Ratcliffe J, Thorpe L, Brazier J, Campbell M, Fitter M, Roman M, Walters S and Nicholl JP. Longer term clinical and economic benefits of offering acupuncture care to patients with chronic low back pain. *Health Technol Asses* 2005; **9**(32): iii-iv, ix-x, 1–109.

16. Tsui MLK, Cheing GLY. The effectiveness of electroacupuncture versus electrical heat acupuncture in the management of chronic low-back pain. *J Alter Complement Med* 2004; **10**(5): 803–809.

17. João Bosco Guerreiro da Silva, Mary Uchiyama Nakamura, José Antonio Cordeiro, Luiz Kulay Jr. Acupuncture for low back pain in pregnancy — a prospective, quasi-randomised, controlled study. *Acupunct Med* 2004; **22**(2): 60–67.

18. Kvorning N, Holmberg C, Grennert L, Aberg A, Akeson J. Acupuncture relieves pelvic and low-back pain in late pregnancy. *Acta Obstetricia et Gynecologica Scandinavica* 2004; **83**(3): 246–250.

19. Meng CF, Wang D, Ngeow J, Lao L, Peterson M, Paget S, Acupuncture for chronic low back pain in older patients: a randomized, controlled trial. *Rheumatology* 2003; **42**(12): 1508–1517.

20. Kerr DP, Walsh DM, Baxter D, Acupuncture in the management of chronic low back pain: a blinded randomized controlled trial. *Clin J Pain* 2003; **19**(6): 364–370

21. Yeung CK, Leung MC, Chow DH, The use of electro-acupuncture in conjunction with exercise for the treatment of chronic low-back pain. *J Alter Complement Med* 2003; **9**(4): 479–490.

22. Giles LG, Muller R, Chronic spinal pain: a randomized clinical trial comparing medication, acupuncture, and spinal manipulation. *Spine* 2003; **28**(14): 1490–1502.

23. Tsukayama H. Yamashita H. Amagai H. Tanno Y. Randomised controlled trial comparing the effectiveness of electroacupuncture and TENS for low back pain: a preliminary study for a pragmatic trial. *Acupunct Med.* 2002; **20**(4): 175–180.

24. Molsberger AF, Mau J, Pawelec DB, Winkler J. Does acupuncture improve the orthopedic management of chronic low back pain — a randomized, blinded, controlled trial with 3 months follow up. *Pain* 2002; **99**(3): 579–587.

25. Ceccherelli F, Rigoni MT, Gagliardi G, Ruzzante L, Comparison of superficial and deep acupuncture in the treatment of lumbar myofascial pain: a double-blind randomized controlled study. *Clin J Pain* 2002; **18**(3): 149–153.

26. Leibing E, Leonhardt U, Koster G, Goerlitz A, Rosenfeldt JA, Hilgers R, Ramadori G. Acupuncture treatment of chronic low-back pain — a randomised, blinded, placebo-controlled trial with 9-month follow-up. *Pain* 2002; **96**(1–2): 189–196.

27. Carlsson CP, Sjolund BH. Acupuncture for chronic low back pain: a randomized placebo-controlled study with long-term follow-up. *Clin J Pain* 2001; **17**(4): 296–305.

28. Kalauokalani D, Cherkin DC, Sherman KJ, Koepsell TD, Deyo RA. Lessons from a trial of acupuncture and massage for low back pain: patient expectations and treatment effects. *Spine* 2001; **26**(13): 1418–1424.

29. Cherkin DC, Eisenberg D, Sherman KJ, Barlow W, Kaptchuk TJ, Street J, Deyo RA. Randomized trial comparing traditional Chinese medical acupuncture, therapeutic massage, and self-care education for chronic low back pain. *Arch Int Med* 2001; **161**(8): 1081–1088.

30. Wedenberg K, Moen B, Norling A. A prospective randomized study comparing acupuncture with physiotherapy for low-back and pelvic pain in pregnancy. *Acta Obstetricia et Gynecologica Scandinavica* 2000; **79**(5): 331–335.

31. Wang RR, Tronnier V. Effect of acupuncture on pain management in patients before and after lumbar disc protrusion surgery — a randomized control study. *Am J Chin Med* 2000; **28**(1): 25–33.

32. Giles LG, Muller R. Chronic spinal pain syndromes: a clinical pilot trial comparing acupuncture, a nonsteroidal anti-inflammatory drug, and spinal manipulation. *J Manip Physiol Ther* 1999; **22**(6): 376–381.

33. Thomas M, Lundberg T. Importance of modes of acupuncture in the treatment of chronic nociceptive low back pain. *Acta Anaesthesiologica Scandinavica* 1994; **38**(1): 63–69.

34. Kitade T, Odahara Y, Shinohara S, Ikeuchi T, Sakai T, Morikawa K, Minamikawa M, Toyota S, Kawachi A, Hyodo M, *et al.* Studies on the enhanced effect of acupuncture analgesia and acupuncture anesthesia by D-phenylalanine (2nd report) — schedule of administration and clinical effects in low back pain and tooth extraction. *Acupunct Electro* 1990; **15**(2): 121–135.

35. Hackett GI, Seddon D, Kaminski D. Electroacupuncture compared with paracetamol for acute low back pain. *Practitioner* 1988; **232**(1443): 163–164.

36. Lehmann TR, Russell DW, Spratt KF Colby H, Liu YK, Fairchild ML, Christensen S. Efficacy of electroacupuncture and TENS in the rehabilitation of chronic low back pain patients. *Pain* 1986; **26**(3): 277–290.

37. Martelete M, Fiori AM. Comparative study of the analgesic effect of transcutaneous nerve stimulation (TNS); electroacupuncture (EA) and meperidine in the treatment of postoperative pain. *Acupunct Electro* 1985; **10**(3): 183–193.

38. Lehmann TR, Russell DW, Spratt KF. The impact of patients with nonorganic physical findings on a controlled trial of transcutaneous electrical nerve stimulation and electroacupuncture. *Spine* 1983; **8**(6): 625–634.

39. Macdonald AJ, Macrae KD, Master BR. Rubin AP. Superficial acupuncture in the relief of chronic low back pain. *Ann Roy Coll Surg* 1983; **65**(1): 44–46.

40. Mendelson G, Selwood TS, Kranz H, Loh TS, Kidson MA, Scott DS. Acupuncture treatment of chronic back pain. A double-blind placebo-controlled trial. *Am J Med* 1983; **74**(1): 49–55.

41. Coan RM, Wong G, Ku SL, Chan YC, Wang L, Ozer FT, Coan PL. The acupuncture treatment of low back pain: a randomized controlled study. *Am J Chin Med* 1980. **8**(1–2): 181–189

42. Gunn CC, Milbrandt WE, Little AS, Mason KE. Dry needling of muscle motor points for chronic low-back pain: a randomized clinical trial with long-term follow-up. *Spine* 1980; **5**(3): 279–291.

43. Zhuang Z, Jiang G. Thirty cases of the blood-stasis type prolapse of lumbar intervertebral disc treated by acupuncture at the Xi (cleft) point plus herbal intervention injection. *J Tradit Chin Med* 2008; **28**(3): 178–182.

44. Sherman KJ, Cherkin DC. Developing methods for acupuncture research: rationale for and design of a pilot study evaluating the efficacy of acupuncture for chronic low back pain. *Altern Ther Health Med* 2003; **9**(5): 54–60.

45. Moher D, Jones A, Lepage L, CONSORT Group. Use of the CONSORT statement and quality of reports of randomized trial: a comparative before-and- after evaluation. *JAMA* 2001, **285**(15): 1992–1995.

46. Mohe RD, Schulz KF, Altman DG. The CONSORT statement: revised recommendations for improving the quality of reports of parallel-group randomised trials. *Lancet* 2001; **357**(9263): 1191–1194.

47. DerSimonian R, Charette LJ, McPeek B, *et al*. Reporting on methods in clinical trials. *N Engl J Med* 1982; **306**(22): 1332–1337.

48. Soares HP, Daniels S, Kumar A, *et al* . Bad reporting does not mean bad methods for randomised trials: observational study of randomised controlled trials performed by the Radiation Therapy Oncology Group. *Brit Med J* 2004; **328**(7430): 22–24.

49. Bian ZX, Li YP, Moher D, *et al*. Improving the quality of randomized controlled trials in Chinese herbal medicine, Part I: clinical trial design and methodology. *Zhong Xi Yi Jie He Xue Bao* 2006; **4**(2): 120–129.

50. Bian ZX, Moher D, DAGENAIS. Improving the quality of randomized controlled trials in Chinese herbal medicine, Part II: control group design. *Zhong Xi Yi Jie He Xue Bao* 2006; **4**(2): 130–136.
51. Bian ZX, Moher D, Dagenais S, *et al*. Improving the quality of randomized controlled trials in Chinese herbal medicine. Part IV: applying a revised CONSORT checklist to measure reporting quality. *Zhong Xi Yi Jie He Xue Bao*, 2006; **4**(3): 233–242
52. MacP H, W Bite A, MIKE CUMMINGS, M.B., Ch.B, Dip.Med.Ac., KIM A. JOBST, KEN ROSE,and RICHARD C. NIEMTZOW. Standards for reporting interventions in controlled. Trials of acupuncture: The STRICTA recommendations. *J Alter Complement Med* 2002; **8**(1), 85–89.
53. Gerhard Fortwengel. *Guide for Clinical Trial Staff Implementing Good Clinical Practice*. Switzerland: K Arger. 2004: p. 74.

CHAPTER 11

ACUPUNCTURE TREATMENT FOR ADDICTION

Ping-Chung Leung,* Ellie S. Y. Pang,*
Lang Zhang* and Eliza L. Y. Wong[†]
*Institute of Chinese Medicine
[†]School of Public and Primary Care
The Chinese University of Hong Kong
5/F, School of Public Health Building
Prince of Wales Hospital, Shatin, Hong Kong

Abstract

A literature review of acupuncture treatment for withdrawal symptoms of heroin addicts showed very positive results. Acupressure on the external ear was also shown to have alleviating effects for chronic smokers determined to quit smoking.

ACUPUNCTURE FOR HEROIN ADDICTION

Opium or heroin dependence has remained the most serious self-destructive addiction all over the world. The usually complicated psycho-social background contributing towards heroine addiction significantly affects the efficacy of popular methods of treatment, none of which offers guaranteed success. With this general lack of standard treatment, acupuncture has been applied as the sole treatment or supplementary offer. A thorough review of the past reports in literature will be useful for the consideration of future application or research.

Review on Clinical Reports about the Use of Acupuncture for Heroine/Opium Addicts

Acupuncture is well-known to be suitable for the control of pain and some autonomic symptoms like nausea, vomiting and dizziness. In China, the application of acupuncture for opium withdrawal is therefore a logical historical attempt. In fact even outside China, for difficult pain related conditions, acupuncture as a treatment option is increasing in popularity. In 1998, the National Institutes of Health of the US held a Consensus Conference which endorsed acupuncture as the therapeutic measure to be recommended for pain, as well as nausea and vomiting control.[1]

Looking through the available literature from 1976 to 2006, more than 70 clinical trials on the use of acupuncture for heroin addiction have been published in the Chinese and English language journals, involving more than 5000 cases.[2] Summarizing the reports about the results of treatment, the suggestions include the following:

(1) Acupuncture gives rapid and efficient effects against the withdrawal symptoms when used as a detoxification agent.[3]
(2) Acupuncture works well together with Methadone in the MMT scheme.[4]
(3) The newer form of auricular acupuncture shows good responses.[5]
(4) Herbal medicine can be used together with acupuncture to give additional effects and acupuncture has better individual effect when compared with the use of herbal medicine alone.[6]
(5) A special meridian and acupuncture points have been identified as particularly suitable for withdrawal therapy.[7]
(6) Electrical stimulation in acupuncture might give better results.[8]
(7) Acupuncture is found to be useful not only as a detoxificating agent, but it might help in preventing relapses.[9]

An analysis of the acupuncture meridian and acupoints used is useful. The following should be noted:

(1) Most acupoints used fell within the *Du Mai* channel (24%), Urinary bladder chanel (15%) and *Ren Mai* channel (9%).
(2) Commonly used body acupoints included:
Neignan (PC 6), *Zusanli* (ST 36), *Hegu* (LI 4), *Sanyinjiao* (SP 6), *Laogong* (PC 8), *Shemen* (HT 7), *Waignan* (SJ 5), *Shenshu* (BL 23), *Baihui* (DU 20), and *Dazhui* (DU I4).
(3) Commonly used auricular acupoints included:
Liver, Kidney, Endocrine, Lung, Heart, Brainstem, usually together with body points. Auricular points were either punctured with short needles which could be retained. Alternatively, small hard beads could be taped onto the ear-lobe for self-pressure manipulations.[9]
(4) Duration of puncture varied from 15 to 60 minutes.

ACUPRESSURE FOR QUITTING CIGARETTE SMOKING

Habitual smoking is relatively harmless compared with heroine addiction. Yet it is becoming a social stigma now that the public is against smokers contaminating the clean environment. The authors are going to offer their own experience conducting a self-administered acupressure clinical trial for the support of quitting smoking.

Review on Clinical Reports about Acupuncture/Acupressure for Quitting Smoking

The smoking cessation study was approved by the Clinical Research Ethics Committee of the Chinese University of Hong Kong. All participants were required to give written informed consent before the trial started. The blocked randomization scheme was used to allocate participants in equal proportions to the active treatment or sham groups. Participants were recruited from outpatient clinics and the community through poster advertisements. Eligible individuals had to be aged

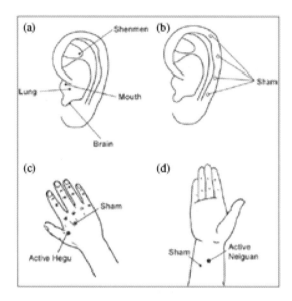

Fig. 1. (A) Active auricular points. (B) Sham auricular points. (C) Active Hegu and sham point. (D) Active Neiguan and sham point.

18 years or older, have a daily cigarette smoking habit, and be motivated to quit smoking. They could not use other smoking cessation therapy simultaneously.

Auricular acupressure was introduced via hard beads fixed with adhesive against the selected acupoints to provide continuous stimulation. Four acupoints on the external ear — *Shenmen*, Lung, Mouth, and Brain — were used.[10] In addition, two more acupoints on the hand — *Hegu* and *Neiguan* — were similarly taped with hard beads. For the sham group, non-specific non-meridian points were chosen away from those selected for the treatment group (Fig. 1 shows the positions of the acupoints).

Participants were instructed to press on the beads repeatedly at least three times a day or whenever they desired to smoke during the three weeks of treatment. They were then followed up weekly during the treatment period, seven days after treatment was completed, and three months after treatment via phone interview.

This pilot study sought to determine whether auricular acupressure could be an effective anti-smoking intervention and if it could help with the relief of withdrawal symptoms. Although there was a lack of statistical evidence to support the efficacy of the active treatment, both active and sham groups revealed a large reduction in the number of cigarettes consumed, confirmed by a substantial reduction of the carbon monoxide level in the breathing tests.

In conclusion, acupressure on the external auricle is a simple maneuver and taking acupoints and sham points together, the positive results reached promising levels. Acupressure is a safe technique for all smokers who want to quit smoking, including pregnant and breastfeeding women, while nicotine replacement therapy might not be as safe and acceptable. Acupressure as a means to help stop smoking may therefore be recommended as a valid option.

REFERENCES

1. National Institutes of Health (NIH), *NIH Public* 1997; **15**(5): 1–34.

2. M. Xu, PhD thesis, Hong Kong: Baptist University, 2007.

3. Montazeri K, Farahnakian M, Saghaei M. *Acta Anaesthesiol Sin* 2002; **40**(4): 173–177.

4. Song X.G, H. Zhang, Z.H. Wang, *et al.*, *Chin. Acup. Mox.* 2002; **12**(12): 795–797.

5. Wang Z.T, Yuan Y.Q, Wang J, Luo J.K, *Shanghai J Acup Mox* 2005; **24**(12), 6–7.

6. Zong L, Hu J, Li Y, Lu Y, Xin Y.F, *Shanghai J Acup Mox* 2001; **20**(2): 1–3.

7. Zeng X.L, Lei L.M, Lu Y.H, Wang Z.T, *Chin. Acup. Mox* 2004; **24**(6): 385–387.

8. Wu L.Z, Cui C.L, Han J.H, *Chin. J. Drug Depend* 2001; **10**(2): 124–126.

9. Shu R, Wen X.Y, Ru L.Q, *et al.*, *Chin. Acup. Mox* 2003; **23**(6): 325–328.

10. Tian Z.M, Chu Y.W, *J Chin Med* 1996; **52**: 5–6.

CHAPTER 12

DENSE CRANIAL ELECTROACUPUNCTURE STIMULATION FOR NEUROPSYCHIATRIC DISORDERS: RATIONALE AND CLINICAL APPLICATION

Zhang-Jin Zhang and Sui-Cheung Man

School of Chinese Medicine, LKS Faculty of Medicine
The University of Hong Kong, Hong Kong, China
zhangzj@hku.hk

Abstract

Dense cranial electroacupuncture stimulation (DCEAS) is a novel stimulation mode in which electrical stimulation is delivered on dense acupoints located on the forehead mainly innervated by the trigeminal nerve. Neuroanatomical evidence suggests that, compared to the spinal-supraspinal pathways, the trigeminal sensory pathway has much intimate connections with the brainstem reticular formation, particularly the dorsal raphe nucleus (DRN) and the locus coeruleus (LC), both of which are the major resources of serotonergic (5-HT) and noradrenergic neuronal bodies, respectively, and play a pivotal role in the regulation of sensation, emotion, sleep, and cognition processing. This has led us to assume that direct stimulation on forehead acupoints in the trigeminal territory could more efficiently produce therapeutic response in neuropsychiatric disorders. Several pilot studies have shown the benefit of DCEAS and similar interventions in patients with headache, refractory obsessive-compulsive disorder (OCD), postpartum depression, and insomnia. Most recently, we have further demonstrated the effectiveness of DCEAS as an additional therapy in the early phase of the treatment of major depression. This paper will discuss related rationale for DCEAS and report the results of our several clinical studies of DCEAS in patients with various neuropsychiatric disorders.

INTRODUCTION

Modern acupuncture can be defined as a therapeutic technique in which sharp, thin needles are inserted into specific points on the body with mechanical, electrical, or other physical stimulation. The nomenclature and localization of most specific points, known as acupuncture points or acupoints, were established in traditional Chinese medicine (TCM) during about B.C. 400–A.D. 1740s. Over the past four decades, numerous clinical observations and studies have shown that acupuncture therapy possesses broad therapeutic benefit.[1,2] A large body of experimental evidence obtained in animals and human subjects provides many insights into neural mechanisms of acupuncture effects, in particular acupuncture analgesia.[3] Today, this ancient healing technique is increasingly introduced into clinical practice, particularly for neuropsychiatric disorders.[2]

Metaphysical Concepts of Acupoint and Meridian in TCM

The doctrine of TCM was originally developed from elementary anatomical knowledge obtained in early days.[4] This is evidenced in numerous gross anatomical studies with measurement and a vast number of anatomical terms recorded in ancient TCM bibliographies. Ancient doctors had observed peripheral nerve trunks, branches, and plexus widely distributed in the superficial and deep tissues as well as on visceral organs, referring to as "meridians" and "collaterals" (*Jing* and *Luo* in Chinese). They believed that the meridians with the collaterals constitute an extensive network that communicates all parts of the body via the meridian energy (*Jing-Qi* in Chinese). The meridian energy can flow onto specific loci, termed 'convergences' or 'conjunctions' in ancient terms and 'acupoints' today. The doctrine of TCM clearly states that acupoints are not the skin, muscles, connective tissues, or bones, but local sites where the meridian energy effuses onto the superficial tissues and infuses into the deep tissues and visceral organs.[4] Ancient doctors also had observed that pathological conditions occurred in the deep tissues and visceral organs can be manifested as pain or tender points on the body, called *A-Shi* points. The localizations and clinical indications for most meridian-based acupoints were initially developed from *A-Shi* points. Ancient doctors suggested that stagnation of the meridian energy is a determining factor in the pathogenesis of diseases. Needling, moxibustion, and other forms of stimulation on acupoints were considered to improve pathological conditions by unblocking the stagnation of the meridian energy and rearranging the balance of Yin and Yang, that is, homeostasis. It would seem that the metaphysical concepts of acupoint and meridian represent an entity with particular anatomical and physiological neural profiles. Nevertheless, how to precisely elucidate the metaphysical concepts of acupoint and meridian in the framework of modern biomedical knowledge has been a key issue in acupuncture research.

"Specific" and "Nonspecific" Properties of Acupoints

As acupoints are deemed 'specific' points in the doctrine of TCM, many efforts have been made to identify their 'specific' properties. Potential differences between the traditionally defined acupoints and so-called "non-acupoints" have been examined at anatomical, istological, biochemical, and electrophysiological levels in both animals and human subjects.[4] Although early studies indicate that most acupoints are located on or adjacent to peripheral nerve trunks or branches, and the meridians correspond with trajectories of relevant peripheral nerve,[4] there is no convincing evidence to support the existence of novel or special structures beneath acupoints. However, histological studies indeed have revealed a relatively dense and concentrated distribution of certain neural and neuroactive components beneath many acupoints commonly used in clinical practice compared to adjacent areas.[4] Electrophysiological studies also have shown that the skin along with acupoints and meridians may possess distinct electrical properties which are closely associated with the activity of local neural and neuroactive components.[5] These results suggest the relativity of the 'specific' and 'non-specific' properties of acupoints. The definition and identification of the pattern of 'specific' and 'non-specific' neural and neuroactive components in the response to acupuncture stimulation would help us better understand the essential mechanisms of acupuncture and develop more efficient acupuncture stimulation modes. However, the metaphysical concept of acupoint and meridian itself cannot provide sufficient information for defining and identifying the response pattern. Interactions between neural and neuroactive components as well as the relationship with the local and central response to acupuncture stimulation are also not well elucidated. Thus, it was necessary to introduce an alternative concept that substantially differentiates from the metaphysical concept of acupoint. Such concept would provide a more accurate term and a new theoretical approach to interpreting effects and mechanisms of acupuncture.

NEURAL ACUPUNCTURE UNIT (NAU)

The Definition and Its Differentiation from Acupoint

Most recently, we have developed a new concept called neural acupuncture unit (NAU) to differentiate the 'specific' and 'non-specific' properties of acupoints.[6] Insertion into the skin with filiform needles is the most commonly used form of acupuncture stimulation in clinical practice. When a filiform needle is inserted into a designated point on the body and mechanical (manual manipulation) or electrical stimulation is delivered, a variety of neural and neuroactive components are activated. A collection of the activated neural and neuroactive components distributed in the skin, muscle, and connective tissues surrounding the inserted needle is defined as a neural acupuncture unit (NAU). Here, the designated points include not only the traditionally defined acupoints, which are often called as meridian-based acupoints or acupoints in short, but also *A-Shi* points and control points (sometimes called non-acupoints or placebo points) as specifically designated in acupuncture research.

NAU Compositions

NAU is a hypothetical concept that represents the collection of local neural and neuroactive components distributed in the skin, muscle, and connective tissues activated by an acupuncture needle that is inserted into a designated point on the body, and mechanical or electrical stimulation is delivered (Fig. 1). The traditionally defined acupoints could be defined as

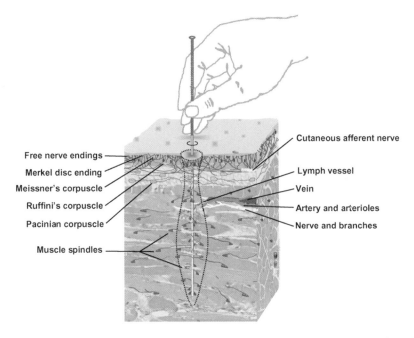

Fig. 1. A representative muscle-spindle-rich NAU in the response to manual twists of acupuncture stimulation. The NAU with the related neural and neuroactive components is illustrated as the dotted line-defined vase-like pattern, which is principally determined by twist produced different distant effects on mechanoreceptors located in cutaneous and muscle tissues.[6]

an anatomical landmark system that indicates local sites where NAUs may contain relatively dense and concentrated neural and neuroactive components, upon which acupuncture stimulation would elicit a more efficient physiological and therapeutic response compared to non-acupoints.

Somatosensory receptors and their afferent fibers are the major neural components of NAUs and play the central role in the production of NAU afferent signals. Neuroactive components of NAUs are non-neuronal tissues and cells that release various mediators capable of modulating NAU afferent signals via local biochemical reactions (Fig. 2).

Biophysical reactions of NAUs are triggered by the activation of mechanoreceptors in NAUs due to mechanical pressure and tissue distortion induced during manual manipulation. NAU-based local mechanism plays an equally important role in acupuncture analgesia as central mechanisms.

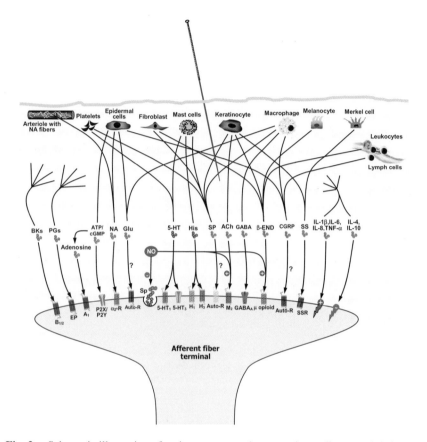

Fig. 2. Schematic illustration of major nonneuronal neuroactivemediators and their corresponding receptors involved in the modulation of NAU afferent impulses. Molecules in red, green, and violet color represent stimulatory, inhibitory, and both effects on afferent fiber excitability, respectively. Autoreceptors to be identified are indicated with question symbols. A1, adenosine A1 receptor; ACh, acetylcholine; Auto-R, autoreceptor; B1/2, bradykinin receptors 1 and 2; BK, bradykinin; CGRP, calcitonin-gene-related peptide; β-END, β-endorphin; EP, prostaglandin E receptor; GABA, γ-aminobutyric acid; Glu, glutamate; H1/H2, histamine H1/H2 receptors; His, histamine; 5-HT, 5-hydroxy-tryptamine; IL, interleukin; M2, muscarinic M2 receptor; NA, noradrenaline; NO, nitric oxide; PG, prostaglandins; P2X/P2Y, purinergic receptors P2X and P2Y; α2-R, α2 adreno-ceptor; SP, substance P; SS, somatostatin; SSR, somatostatin receptor; TNF-α, tumor necrosis factor-α.[6]

Different types of NAUs are associated with different NAU afferent impulses and components of needling sensation. The biochemical and biophysical reactions of NAUs dominantly activate small-diameter (Aδ and C) and myelinated afferent fibers (Aβ and Aδ), respectively. The induction of aching, soreness, and warmth of needling sensation are closely associated with the activation of Aδ and C fibers in NAUs, whereas numbness, heaviness, and distension are mainly related to the activation of Aβ and Aδ fibers.

Based on the predominance of somatosensory receptors, NAUs can be roughly classified into the three types: muscle-spindle-rich NAUs, cutaneous-receptor-rich NAUs, and tendon-organ-rich NAUs. Table 1 summarizes the definition, characteristics, and related acupoints of the three types of NAUs.

Multiple central neural pathways convey NAU afferent impulses. The spinothalamic and spinoreticular tracts dominantly transmit biochemical reaction evoked signals, whereas the dorsal column-medial lemniscus tract mainly transmits mechanoreceptor-activated signals. The trigeminal sensory pathway that conveys NAU afferent signals from the trigeminal

Table 1. The putative relationship between NAU properties and needling.

NAU Properties	Components of Needling Sensation	
	Aching/Soreness/Warmth **Numbness/Heaviness/** **Distension**	
Type of NAUs	Cutaneous receptor-rich NAUs with a predominance of nociceptors.	Muscle spindle- and tendon organ-rich NAUs.
NAU reactions	Biochemical reaction.	Biophysical reaction.
Dominant afferent fibers	Aδ and C.	Aβ and Aδ.
Acupuncture stimulation modes	Prick; shallow needling; high-frequency EA; laser acupuncture' heat acupuncture.	Most manual techniques in gentle and repetitive manipulation; low-frequency, high-intensity EA and TENS.

territory has closer connections with the brainstem reticular formation, particularly 5-HT and catecholaminergic neuronal systems, which play a pivotal role in the modulation of broad effects of acupuncture.

A distributed network of widespread brain regions that respond to acupuncture provides the neural substrate for the broad therapeutic effects of acupuncture. The more widespread and intense brain regional response may be a consequence of more efficient NAU stimulation. A frequency-specific neurochemical response in the CNS may be related to differential response of NAUs to low- and high-frequency EA stimulation and different peripheral and central pathways. Acupuncture has broad effects of normalizing neuroimaging, neurochemical, and behavioral abnormalities in neuropsychiatric disorders as well as regulating autonomic activities in visceral disorders. These effects may be achieved initially by rearranging the subtle balance of neuroactive mediators and modulating NAU afferent impulses.

Implications and Future Directions of NAU

The establishment of the conception of NAU and its differentiation from acupoint not only provide an alternative theoretical approach into acupuncture research, but also bring many implications and impacts on further directions.

Scientific rationale for traditional needling techniques

The NAU-based local mechanism by which acupuncture stimulation locally modulates NAU biochemical reactions provides an important scientific rationale for traditional multiple-needling techniques, such as seven-star needling, plum-blossom-like needling, and round-needling, most of which are specifically used to treat focal lesions and pain conditions. The clarification of differences in local effects between multiple-needling and other needling techniques will help develop more efficient and specific acupuncture treatment regimens. Although the local roles of some NAU neuroactive mediators are well defined in acupuncture analgesia,[7–10] most NAU mediators need to be further examined.

Multiple central neural pathways

While most previous studies have placed the emphasis on the lateral funiculus of the spinal cord, the dorsal column-medial lemniscus tract and the trigeminal sensory pathway have received relatively less attention. As mechanoreceptor-activated signals dominate in most NAU afferent impulses, particularly in muscle-spindle-rich and tendon-organ rich NAUs, the role of the dorsal column-medial lemniscus tract in acupuncture effects deserves to be further clarified. As an efficient stimulation mode, Dense Cranial Electroacupuncture Stimulation (DCEAS) was developed based on the neuroanatomical rationale that NAUs in the trigeminal territory have intimate connections with the brainstem reticular formation. Neurophysiological and neuroimaging studies of this novel acupuncture mode will provide direct evidence to prove its efficiency.

Synergistic effects of multiacupoints

In clinical practice, acupuncture treatment regimens generally consist of multiacupoints located in different parts of the body. Empirical and experimental evidence suggests that the combination of local and distant acupoints produces greater treatment effects than the sum of single acupoints. Different central mechanisms are implicated in processing acupuncture signals from acupoints located in homeo- and heterosegmental spinal nerve territory.[11] Simultaneous stimulation of different acupoints appears to elicit more widespread and intense brain regional response.[12] Given that superior therapeutic response is associated with synergistic or additive effects of NAUs at local and systemic levels, the clarification of this relationship will provide valuable information in the development of more efficient acupuncture treatment regimens.

Explanations to effects of sham acupuncture

Sham acupuncture often serves as a control in basic and clinical acupuncture research. The two most commonly used sham procedures are (1) insertion of acupuncture needles into control points generally defined at a certain distances (usually 1–3 cm) from acupoints and (2) noninserted placebo needling on the same acupoints.[13] These control procedures were initially designed to differentiate specific acupuncture effects at acupoints from nonacupoints. Nevertheless, as mentioned earlier, the most notable difference between most acupoints and non-acupoints is the relatively higher density of certain neural and neuroactive components with pre-dominance and concentration of somatosensory receptors and their afferent fibers in acupoint-based NAUs. Clinically, it might be difficult to differentiate the effects of acupoints from adjacent points; even if needles are not inserted into the skin at nonacupoints, it may excite mechanoreceptors of NAUs. This could, at least in part, explain why most clinical studies have failed to demonstrate superior efficacy in "real" (or called "true", verum or genuine) acupuncture treatment regimens compared to sham or placebo regimens; sham acupuncture intervention even displays superior efficacy compared to inert placebo acupuncture.[1,14] In order to identify the systemic effects of acupuncture, a valid control design should completely block the production of NAU afferent impulses. For this purpose, the utilization of modified needles with local anesthetic drugs might be considered.

Discoveries on objective measures of acupuncture 'dosage'

Inadequate 'dose' is thought to be an important factor in the failure of many clinical studies of acupuncture to achieve positive treatment outcomes.[15] Indeed, our recent meta-analysis of acupuncture therapy in depressive disorders[16] and a systematic review[17] have confirmed that most clinical trials did not include criteria for either qualitative or quantitative adequacy of acupuncture treatment regimens. Acupuncture 'dosage' in fact represents both local and systemic efficiency of NAU stimulation. Local efficiency can be reflected in changes in local NAU-associated biochemical and electrodermal indices; systemic efficiency may be indicated in the needling sensation, neuroimaging, or neurochemical response recorded in CNS. While the verbal report of the intensity of needling sensation as a subjective scale has been demonstrated to be a valid psychological indicator for the intensity of acupuncture stimulation,[18] the exploration of NAU-associated neurophysiological and neurochemical indicators may result in the discovery of objective measures of acupuncture 'dosage.'

DENSE CRANIAL ELECTROACUPUNCTURE STIMULATION

Based on the neuroanatomical rationale that NAUs in the trigeminal territory have intimate connections with the brainstem reticular formation, Dense cranial electroacupuncture stimulation (DCEAS) is developed as a novel stimulation mode in which electrical stimulation is delivered on dense acupoints located on the forehead mainly innervated by the trigeminal nerve, efficiently modulating multiple central transmitter systems via the trigeminal sensory-brainstem NA and 5-HT neuronal pathways (Fig. 3).[19] Several pilot studies have shown that DCEAS and similar approaches are effective in improving refractory obsessive-compulsive disorder (OCD),[19] major depressive disorder (MDD),[20] post-stroke depression,[21] and MDD-associated residual insomnia.[22] To further investigate the effects of DCEAS, we recently performed several clinical studies on patients with various mental disorders, as illustrated below.

DCEAS for Major Depressive Disorder[23]

This was a single blind, randomized, controlled study to determine whether DCEAS intervention could produce greater clinical improvement compared to noninvasive electroacupuncture (n-EA) control procedure in the early phase of selective serotonin reuptake inhibitor (SSRI) treatment of Major Depressive Disorder (MDD). Approved by the Institutional Review Board (IRB) of the University of Hong Kong and research ethics committees (REC) of local hospitals, the study was conducted in the Department of Psychiatry at Kowloon Hospital between August 2009 and March 2011.

Psychiatrists referred outpatients to the study. All participants who met selective criteria gave voluntary, written consent before entering the trial. They were randomly assigned to nine-session DCEAS or non-invasive electroacupuncture (n-EA) control procedure in combination with fluoxetine (FLX) for three weeks. Clinical outcomes were measured using the 17-item Hamilton Depression Rating Scale (HAMD-17), Clinical Global Impressionseverity (CGI-S), and Self-rating Depression Scale (SDS) as well as the response and remission rates.

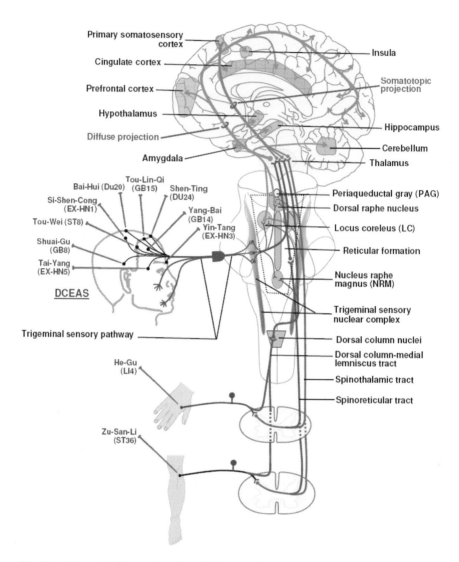

Fig. 3. Schematic illustration of multiple central neural pathways transmitting NAU afferent impulses from different parts of the body. The brain areas commonly observed in neuroimaging response to acupuncture stimulation are indicated with gray shadow. DCEAS: dense cranial electroacupuncture stimulation.[6]

Seventy-three patients were randomly assigned to *n*-EA (*n* = 35) and DCEAS (*n* = 38), of whom 34 in *n*-EA and 36 in DCEAS group were analyzed. DCEAS-treated patients displayed a significantly greater reduction from baseline in HAMD-17 scores at Day 3 through Day 21 and in SDS scores at Day 3 and Day 21 compared to patients receiving *n*-EA. DCEAS intervention also produced a higher rate of clinically significant response compared to *n*-EA procedure (19.4% (7/36) vs. 8.8% (3/34)). The incidence of adverse events was similar in the two groups.

In this study, we found that DCEAS is a safe and effective intervention that augments the antidepressant efficacy. It can be considered as an additional therapy in the early phase of SSRI treatment of depressed patients.

Pilot Trial of DCEAS for Postpartum Depression[24]

This was a randomized, subject- and assessor-blind, parallel-group, sham-controlled trial. Approved by the local institutional review board, the study was conducted at the Department of Obstetrics and Gynaecology in three regional hospitals in Hong Kong, covering approximately half a million population. Subjects were recruited from June 2010 to December 2011, initially in one hospital then extended to three hospitals from February 2011.

Women in the maternity wards 1–3 days postpartum were invited to enroll in the study and participate in a telephone screening for postpartum depression 3–6 weeks after child birth. After given written informed consent, patients meeting selection criteria were randomly assigned to DCEAS or *n*-EA two sessions weekly for four weeks. The assessment of depressive symptoms using the Edinburgh Postnatal Depression Scale (EPDS) and HAMD-17 was performed by independent research assistants and clinicians who were blinded to group allocation. The subjects were assessed by the same clinician at every study visit.

Twenty women within six months postpartum with DSM-IV-diagnosed major depressive disorder of mild severity, defined as a 17-item Hamilton Depression Rating Scale (HAMD-17) score of 12 to 19, joined the study. A significant reduction in HAMD-17 score from baseline to four-week post-treatment was found in both groups, with an effect size 1.37 and 1.80 for DCEAS and *n*-EA, respectively. Improvement was observed as early as two weeks after commencing acupuncture. The response and remission rate in the DCEAS group at four-week posttreatment was 33.3% and 44.4%, respectively; for the *n*-EA group, it was 60.0% and 50.0%, respectively. Except a better work functioning as measured by the Sheehan Disability Scale in the *n*-EA group at immediate post-treatment and four-week posttreatment, there was no significant between-group difference in other outcome measures. Treatment credibility, success of blinding, and adverse events were similar between groups.

The finding in this study provided important data on the management of postpartum major depressive disorder using acupuncture. Further studies utilizing larger sample size and home-based treatment are warranted to accurately determine the efficacy of DCEAS for postpartum depression.

DCEAS for OCD — A Pilot Waitlist-Controlled Trial[19]

A large proportion of obsessive-compulsive disorder (OCD) patients are refractory to pharmacological and cognitive-behavioral therapy. A pilot, waitlist-controlled trial was carried out to evaluate the effectiveness of electroacupuncture (EA) as add-on therapy for treatment-resistant OCD. Approved by the Medical Ethical Committee of First Teaching Hospital of Hebei Medical University, eligible participants with written informed consent were assigned to receive DCEAS treatment for 12 sessions (five sessions per week) or waitlist as controls in nonrandom manner, along with their current anti-OCD medications. The clinical response, defined as $\geq 30\%$ reduction in Yale-Brown Obsessive-Compulsive Scale (YBOCS) score and Clinical Global Impression-Severity (CGI-S) at end point from baseline, was also calculated. Adverse events, reported, elicited or observed, were recorded on case report form, including date and time of onset, duration, severity, relationship to study drug, and action taken.

Nineteen patients with treatment-resistant OCD were assigned to EA treatment for 12 sessions (five sessions per week, $n = 10$) or waitlist for controls ($n = 9$) while continuing their current anti-OCD medications. The clinical outcomes were measured using the YBOCS and the CGI-S at baseline and end point. EA additional treatment produced significantly greater improvements at end point compared with the waitlist group in reducing both YBOCS (10.2 ± 4.2 vs. 18.8 ± 7.4, $p = 0.004$) and CGI-S scores (3.0±1.1 vs. 4.4±1.1, $p = 0.002$). As an additional therapy, DCEAS is effective in alleviating OCD symptoms of treatment-resistant patients. The results from this pilot study warrant a large-scale controlled study.

DCEAS for Post-Stroke Depression (Recruiting)

A large proportion of stroke patients develop post-stroke depression (PSD), either in the early or late stages after stroke. Although antidepressant agents, represented by selective serotonin reuptake inhibitors (SSRIs), are recommended as first-line drugs in pharmaco-therapy of PSD, its effectiveness is limited and the clinical use is largely hampered due to broad side effects, especially on cardiovascular system. In addition, since stroke patients are often medicated with various classes of drugs, the addition of antidepressant agents may increase risk of drug-drug interactions, resulting in unexpected and unpredictable adverse events.

On the hypothesis that DCEAS combined with antidepressants could produce greater therapeutic effects than antidepressants alone, this four-week, assessor-blind, randomized, controlled study of DCEAS as additional treatment with the SSRIs is designed (ClinicalTrials.gov ID: NCT01174394). A total of 60 patients with PSD will be recruited, who will be randomly assigned to FLX (10–30 mg/day) combined with active cranial and body acupuncture ($n = 30$) or FLX with placebo cranial and active body acupuncture ($n = 30$) (12 sessions, three sessions a week). Changes in the severity of depressive symptoms over time are measured using depressive scale instruments. Clinical response and remission rates are also calculated.

A Neuroimaging Study on DCEAS (Recruiting)

As found in previous clinical study that that DCEAS is clinically safe and effective in augmenting the antidepressant efficacy in early SSRI treatment,[23] we hypothesize that the normalizing effect is associated with the modulation of various nervous functions associated with the pathophysiology of MDD. Therefore a neuroimaging study of DCEAS study is designed to delineate the related mechanisms (ClinicalTrials. gov ID: NCT01479920).

In this six-week, assessor-blind, randomized, controlled study of DCEAS as additional treatment with the antidepressant drug FLX, a total of 40 patients with major depressive disorder (MDD) will be recruited. The patients will be randomly assigned to FLX (10–30 mg/day) combined with sham ($n = 41$) or FLX with active DCEAS ($n = 41$) (18 sessions, three sessions a week). Changes in the severity of depressive symptoms over time are measured using depressive instruments. Clinical response and remission rates are also calculated. Two sessions of PET scan and fMRI will be conducted at baseline and endpoint.

ACKNOWLEDGMENTS

This paper was derived from acupuncture research projects supported by Health and Health Services Research Fund (HHSRF) of Hong Kong Food and Health Bureau (Ref. no.: 06070831), General Research Fund (GRF) of Hong Kong Research Grant Council (RGC) (Ref. no.: 786611), HKU intramural funds (Ref. no.: 10400876), Hospital Authority Research Funds, Sir Michael and Lady Kadoorie charitable donation; Natural Science Foundation of China (No. 30870886) and the 11th Five-Year Project of Military Medicine Foundations (2008ZXJ09014-002 and 08Z031). The funding agents had no role in study design, data collection and analysis, preparation of the manuscript, and decision of publication.

REFERENCES

1. Linde K, Vickers A, Hondras M, *et al.* Systematic reviews of complementary therapies — an annotated bibliography. Part 1: acupuncture, *BMC Complem Altern Med* 2001; **1**: 3.
2. Park J, Linde K, Manheimer E, *et al.* The status and future of acupuncture clinical research. *J Altern Complem Med* 2008; **14**(7): 871–881.
3. Zhao ZQ, Neural mechanism underlying acupuncture analgesia, *Prog Neurobiol* 2008; **85**(4): 355–375.
4. Zhou F, Huang D, Xia Y. Neuroanatomical basis of acupuncture points. In: Xia Y, Wu G, Cao X, *et al.* (eds.) *Acupuncture Therapy for Neurological Diseases: A Neurobiological View*, Beijing, China: Tsinghua University Press, 2010: 32–80.

5. Ahn AC, Colbert AP, Anderson BJ, *et al.* Electrical properties of acupuncture points and meridians: a systematic review. *Bioelectromagnetics* 2008; **29**(4): 245–256.

6. Zhang ZJ, Wang XM, McAlonan GM. Neural acupuncture unit: a new concept for interpreting effects and mechanisms of acupuncture. *Evid-Based Compl Alt* 2012; 2012: Article ID 429412.

7. Zhang GG, Yu C, Lee W, Lao L, Ren K, Berman BM. Involvement of peripheral opioid mechanisms in electroacupuncture analgesia. *Explore* 2005; **1**(5): 365–371.

8. Goldman N, Chen M, Fujita T, *et al.* Adenosine A1 receptors mediate local anti-nociceptive effects of acupuncture. *Nature Neurosci* 2010; **13**(7); 883–888.

9. Zhang D, Ding G, Shen X, *et al.* Role of mast cells in acupuncture effect: a pilot study. *Explore* 2008; **4**(3): 170–177.

10. Guan X, Liang X, Liu X. Acetylcholine and the primary input of acupuncture sensation — influence of peripheral acetylcholine on the role of electroacupuncture analgesia. *Zhen Ci Yan Jiu* 1990; **15**(2): 136–139 (Chinese).

11. Bowsher D. Mechanisms of acupuncture. In: Filshie J and White A, eds. *Medical Acupuncture: A Western Scientific Approach*, Edinburgh, UK: Churchill Livingstone, 1998: pp. 69–82.

12. Zhang WT, Jin Z, Luo F, Zhang L, Zeng YW, Han JS. Evidence from brain imaging with fMRI supporting functional specificity of acupoints in humans. *Neurosci Lett* 2004; **354**(1): 50–53.

13. Streitberger K and Kleinhenz J. Introducing a placebo needle into acupuncture research. *Lancet* 1998; **352**(9125): 364–365.

14. Linde K, Niemann K, Schneider A, Meissner K. How large are the nonspecific effects of acupuncture? A meta-analysis of randomized controlled trials. *BMC Med* 2010; **8**: article 75.

15. Benham A Johnson MI. Could acupuncture needle sensation be a predictor of analgesic response? *Acupunct Med* 2009; **27**(2): 65–67.

16. Zhang ZJ, Chen HY, Yip KC, Ng R, Wong VT. The effectiveness and safety of acupuncture therapy in depressive disorders: systematic review and meta-analysis. *J Affect Disorders* 2010; **124**(1–2): 9–21.

17. White A, Cummings M, Barlas P, *et al.* Defining an adequate dose of acupuncture using a neurophysiological approach — a narrative review of the literature. *Acupunct Med* 2008; **26**(2): 111–120.

18. Carlton SM and Coggeshall RE. Immunohistochemical localization of 5-HT(2A) receptors in peripheral sensory axons in rat glabrous skin. *Brain Res* 1997; **763**(2): 271–275.

19. Zhang ZJ, Wang XY, Tan QR, Jin GX, Yao SM. Electroacupuncture for refractory obsessive-compulsive disorder: a pilot waitlist-controlled trial. *J Nerv Ment Dis* 2009; **197**: 619–622.

20. Huang Y, Gong W, Zou J, Zhao CH. An SCL-90 analysis of scalp electroacupuncture treatment of major depressive episode. *Shanghai Zhen Jiu Za Zhi* 2004; **23**: 5–7. (in Chinese with English abstract).

21. Li HJ, Zhong BL, Fan YP, Hu HT. Acupuncture for post-stroke depression: a randomized controlled trial. *Zhongguo Zhen Jiu* 2011; **31**: 3–6. (in Chinese with English abstract).

22. Yeung WF, Chung KF, Tso KC, Zhang SP, Zhang ZJ, *et al.* Electroacupuncture for residual insomnia associated with major depressive disorder: a randomized controlled trial. *Sleep* 2011; **34**: 807–815.

23. Zhang ZJ, Ng R, Man SC, Li TYJ, Wong W, *et al.* Dense cranial electroacupuncture stimulation for major depressive disorder — a single-blind, randomized, controlled study. *PLoS ONE* 2012; **7**(1): e29651.

24. Chung KF, Zhang ZJ, Yeung WF, Lee CP, Ziea E, Wong VT. Randomized non-invasive sham-controlled pilot trial of electroacupuncture for postpartum depression. *J Affect Disorders* 2012(in press).

25. Dhond RP, Kettner N, and Napadow V. Neuroimaging acupuncture effects in the human brain. *J Altern Complem Med* 2007; **13**(6): 603–616.